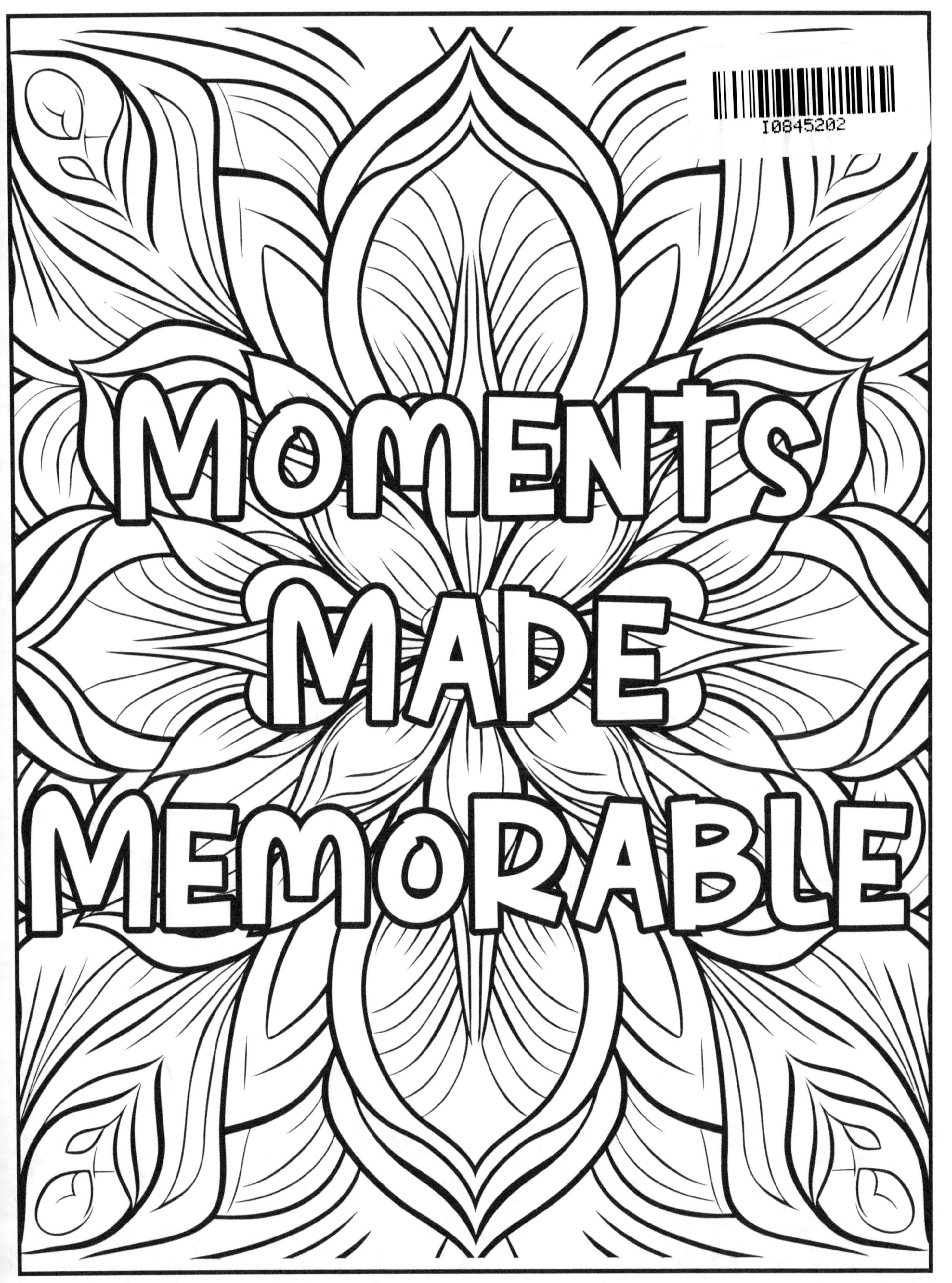

MOMENTS
MADE
MEMORABLE

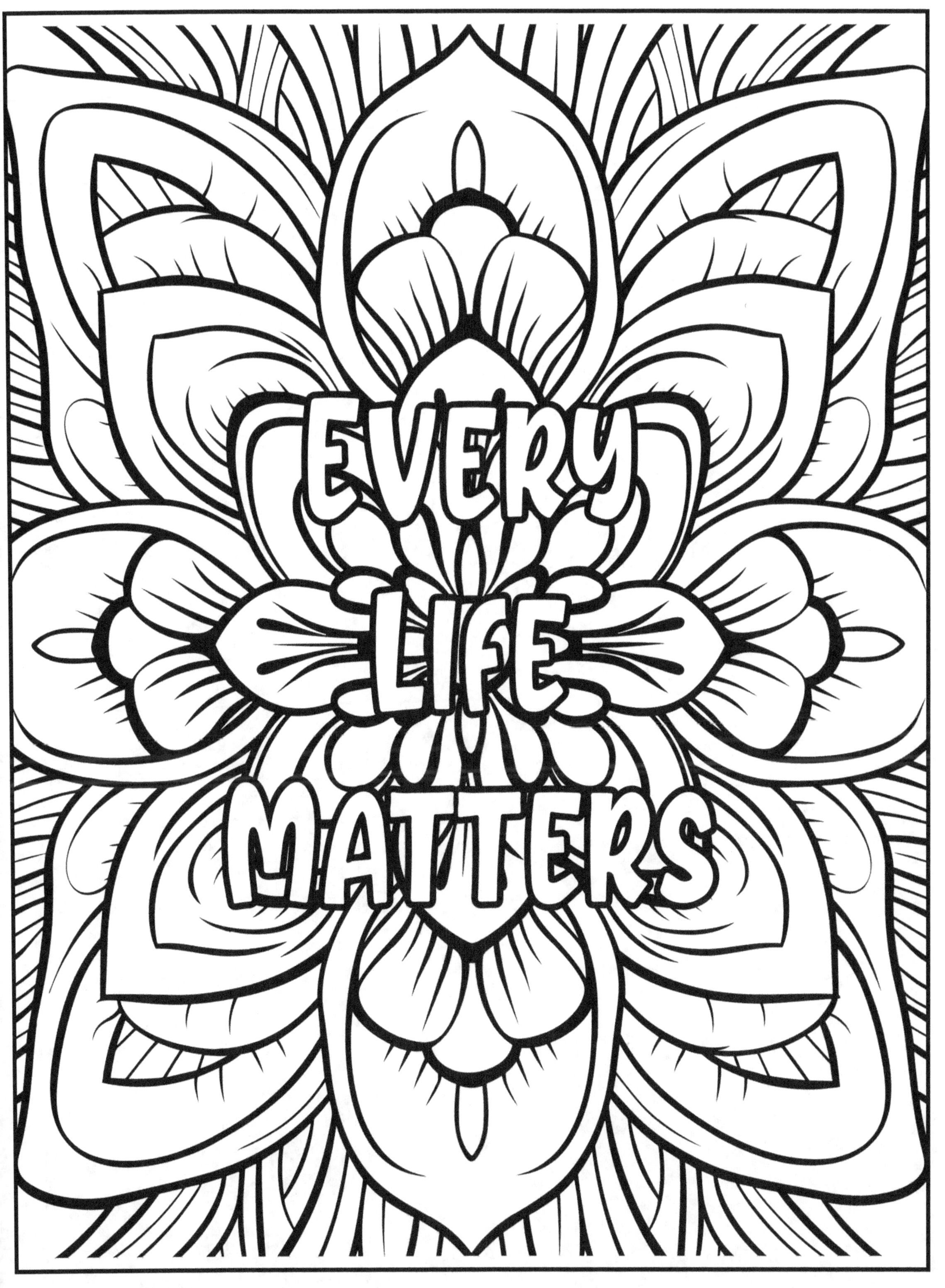

EVERY
LIFE
MATTERS

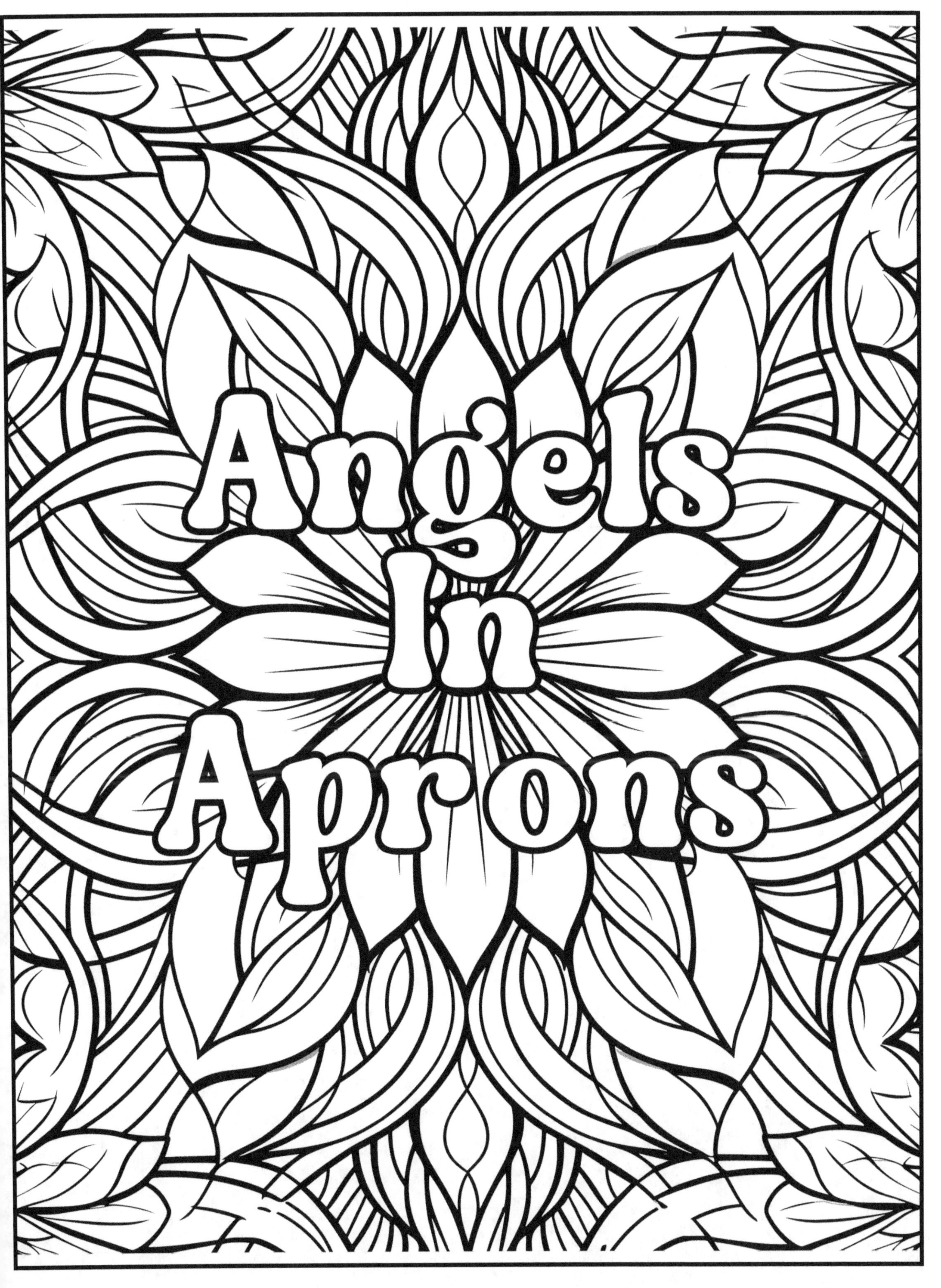

Angels
In
Aprons

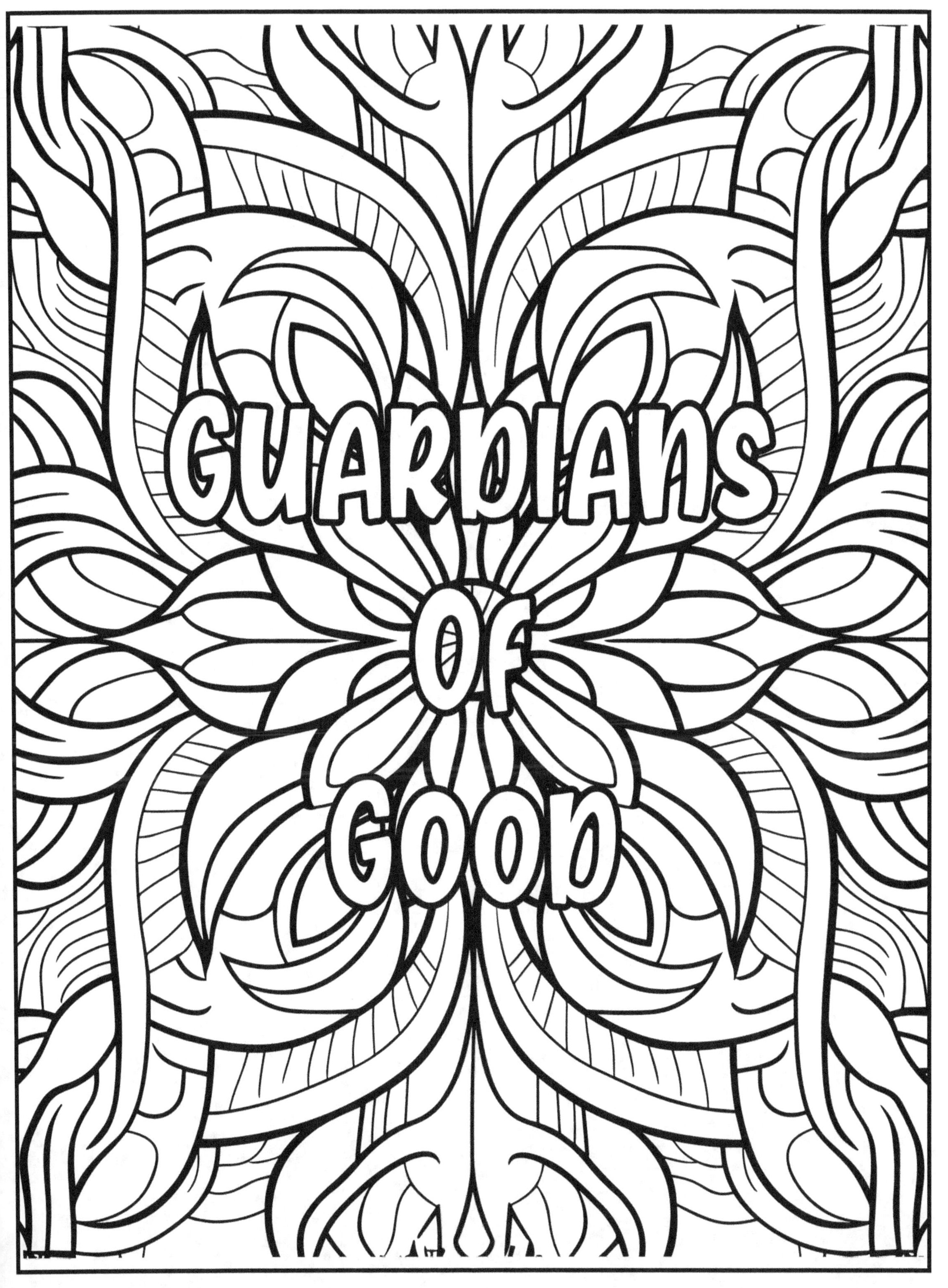

GUARDIANS
OF
GOOD

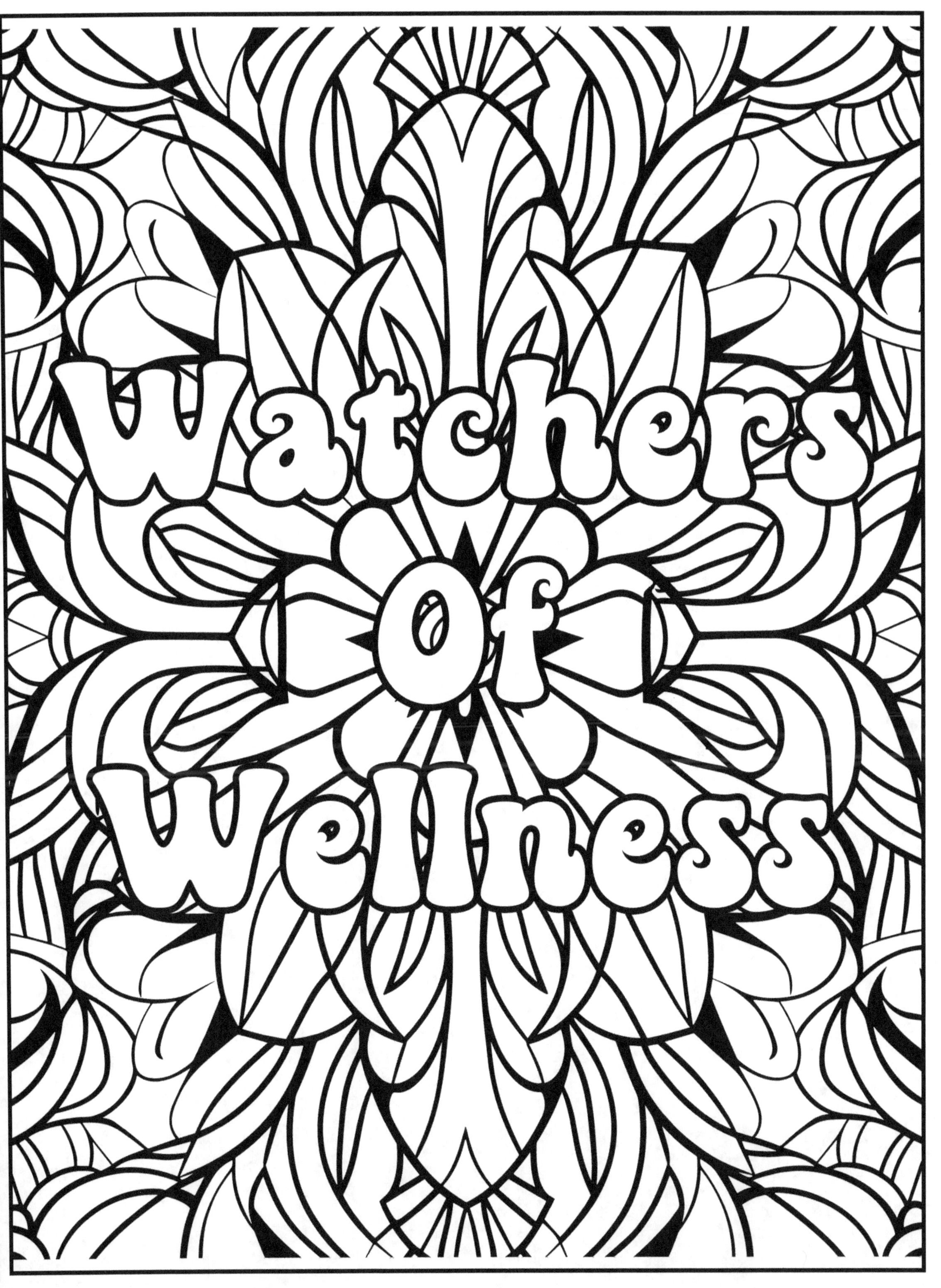
Watchers
Of
Wellness

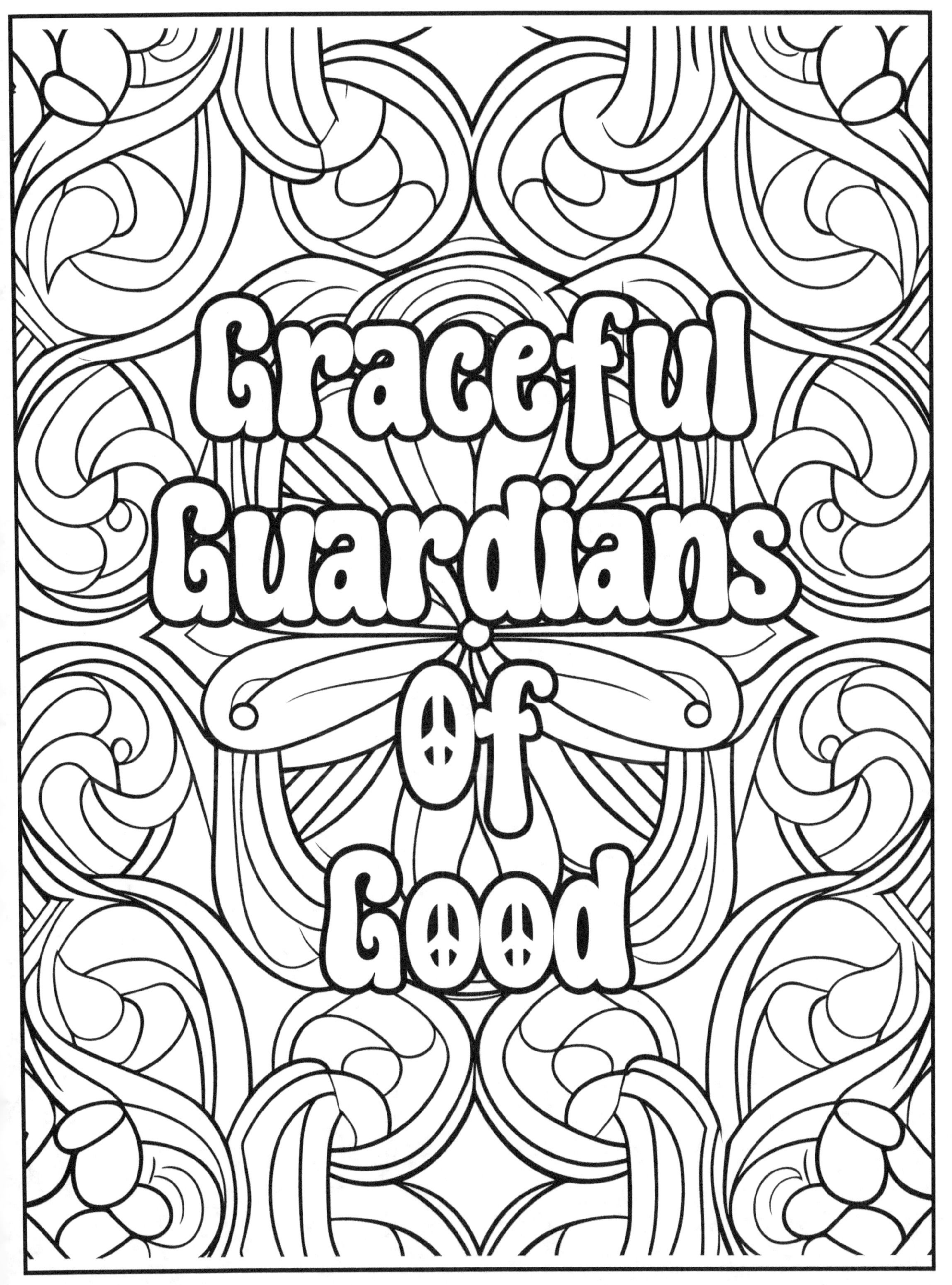

Graceful
Guardians
Of
Good

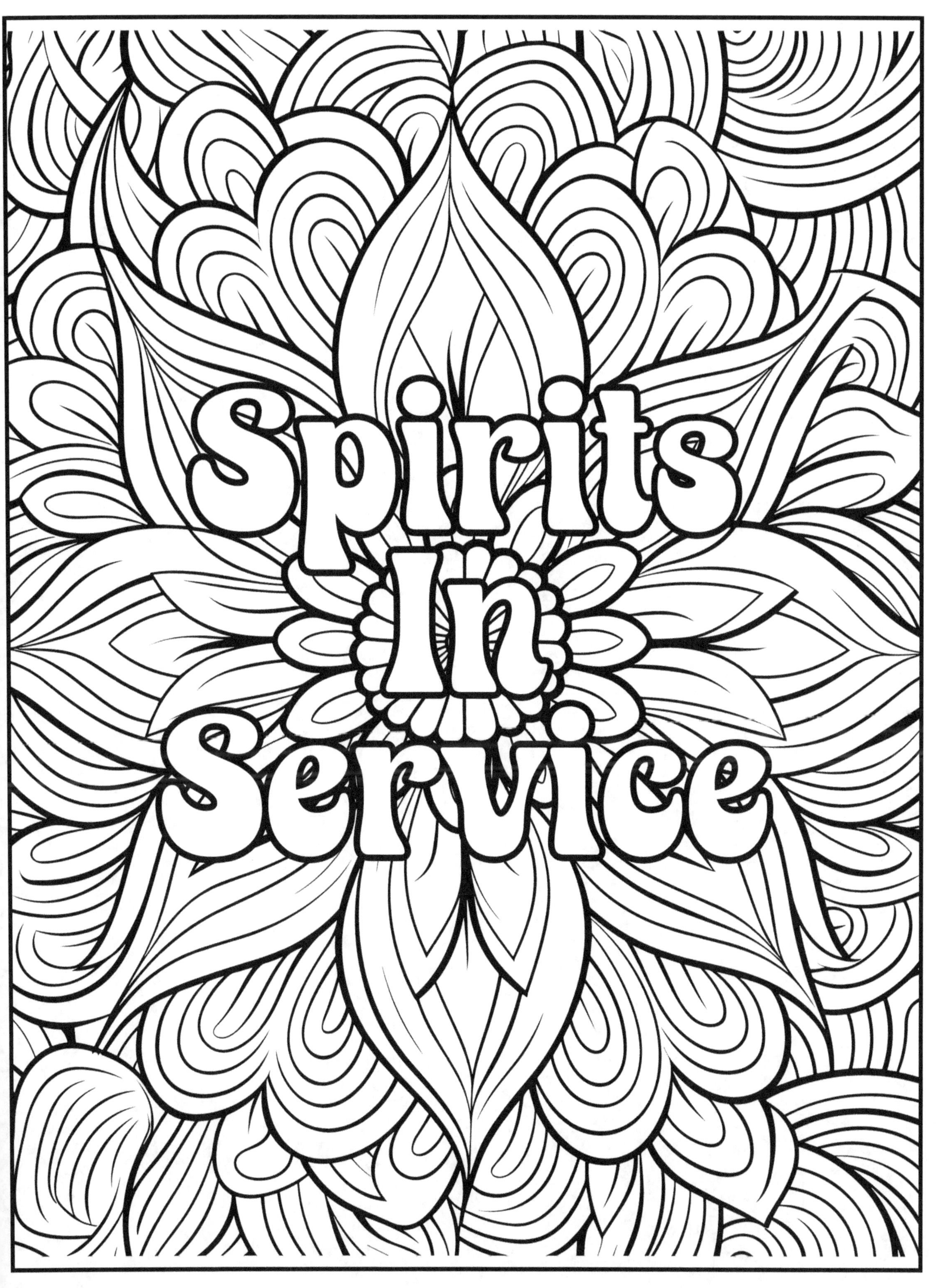
Spirits
In
Service

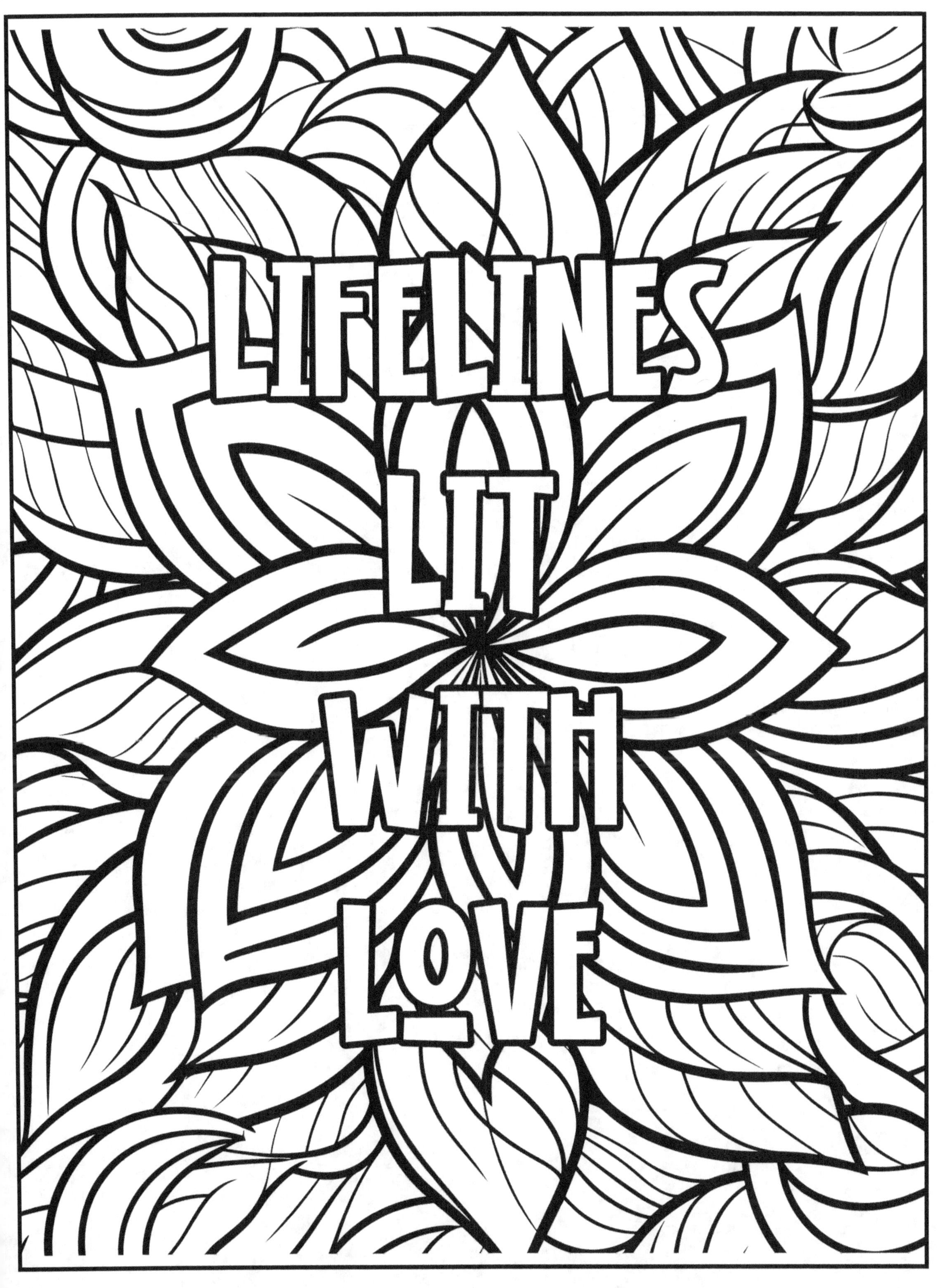

LIFELINES
LIT
WITH
LOVE

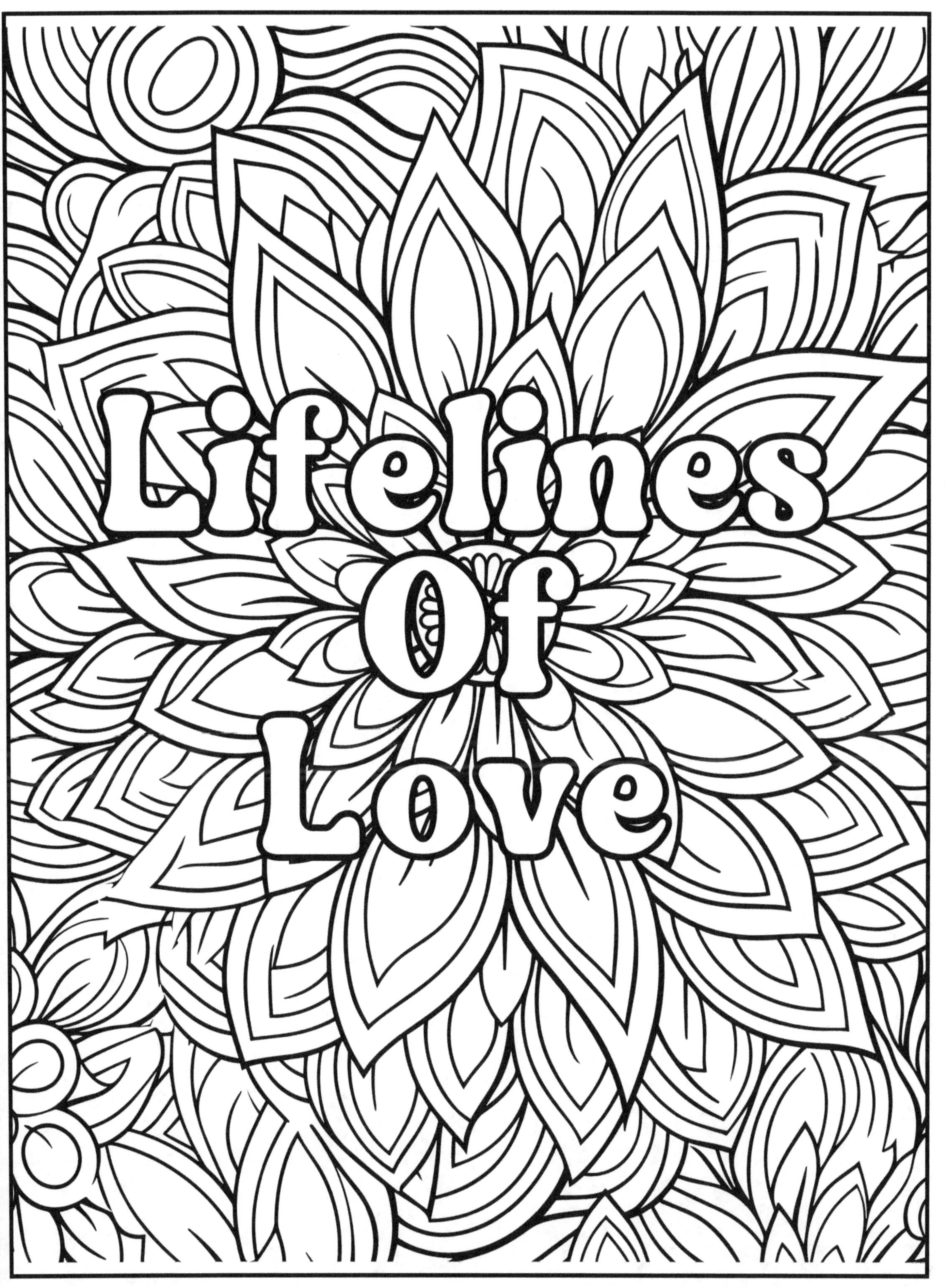
Lifelines
Of
Love

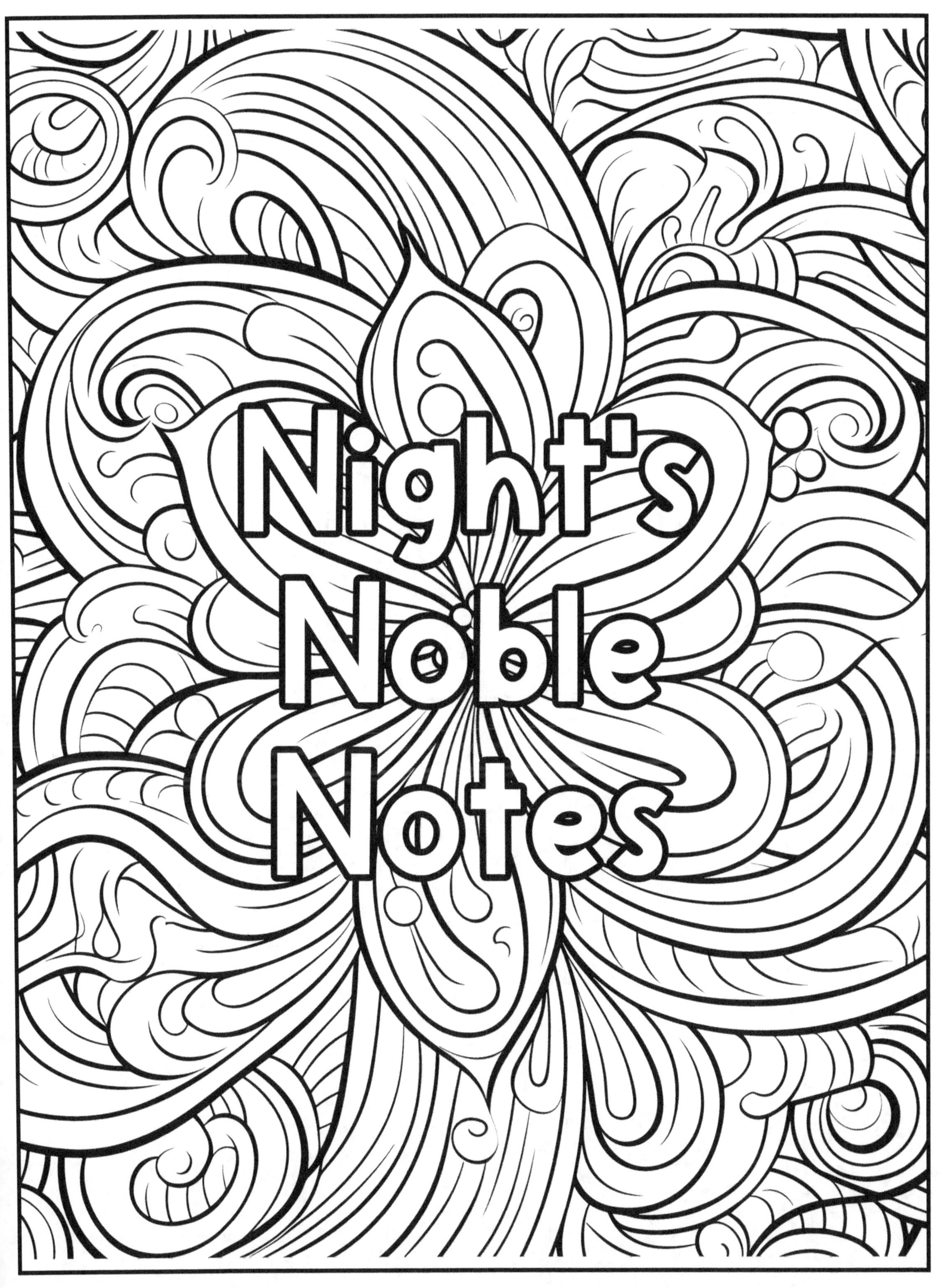
Night's
Noble
Notes

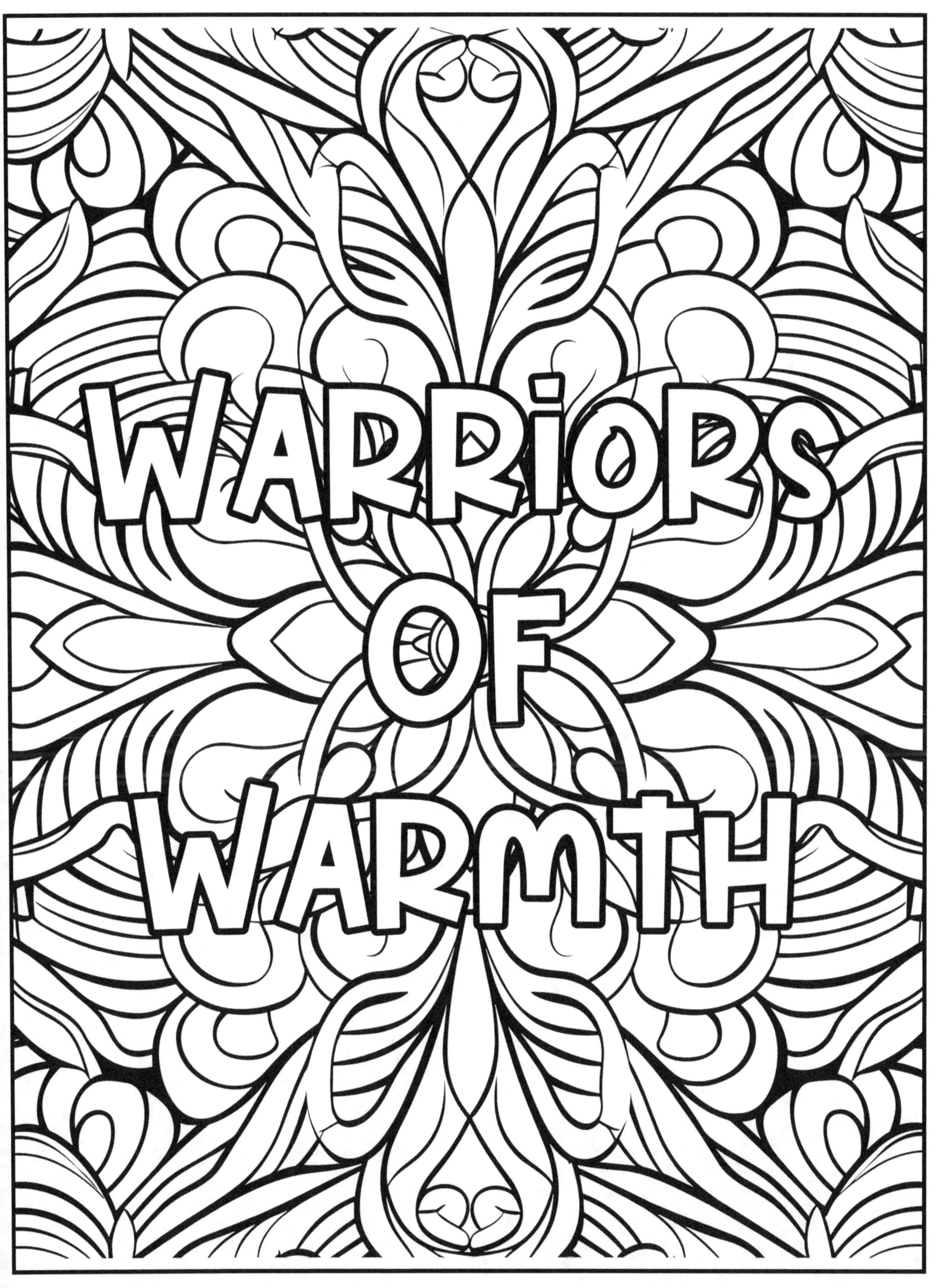

WARRIORS
OF
WARMTH

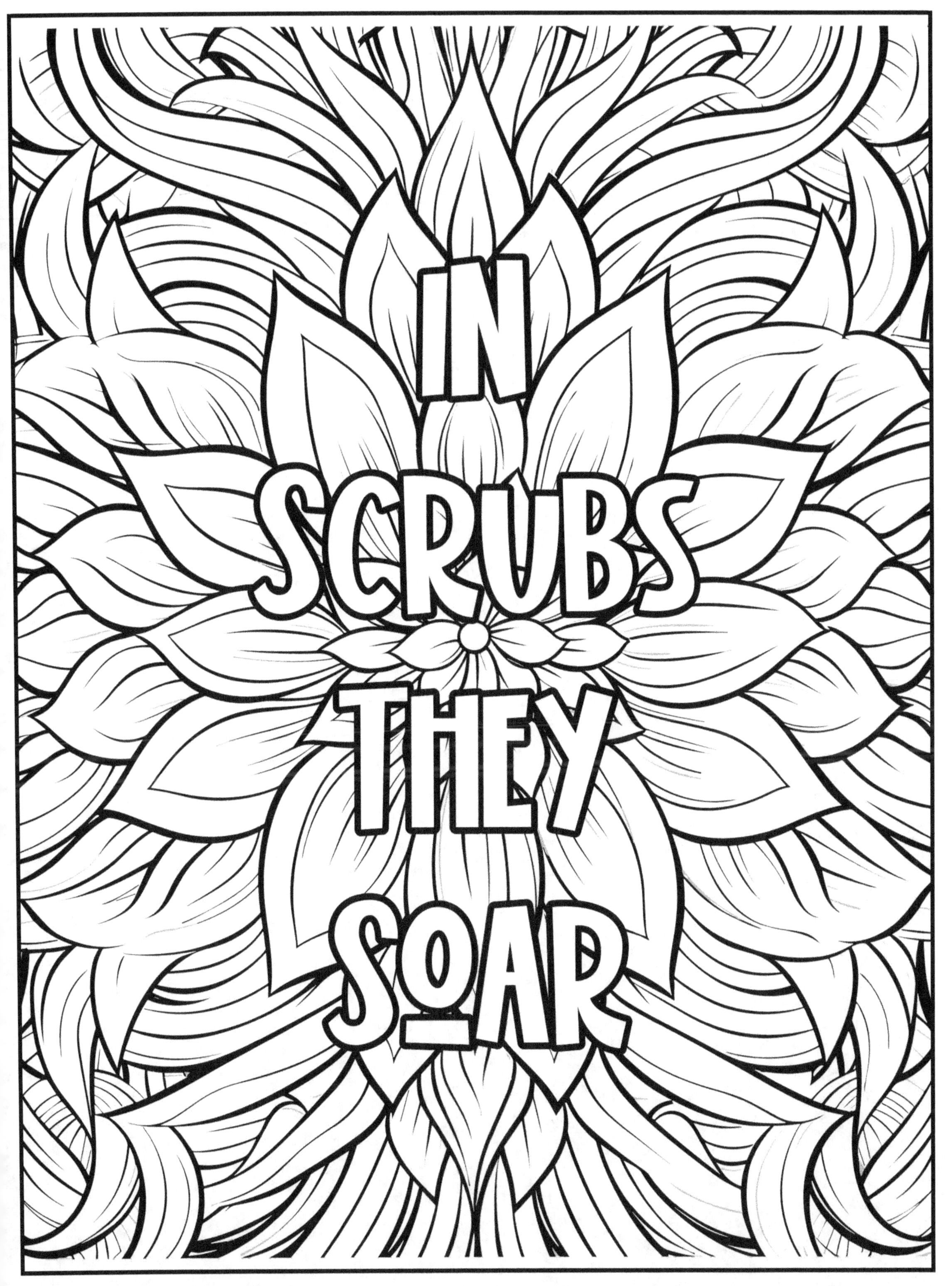

IN
SCRUBS
THEY
SOAR

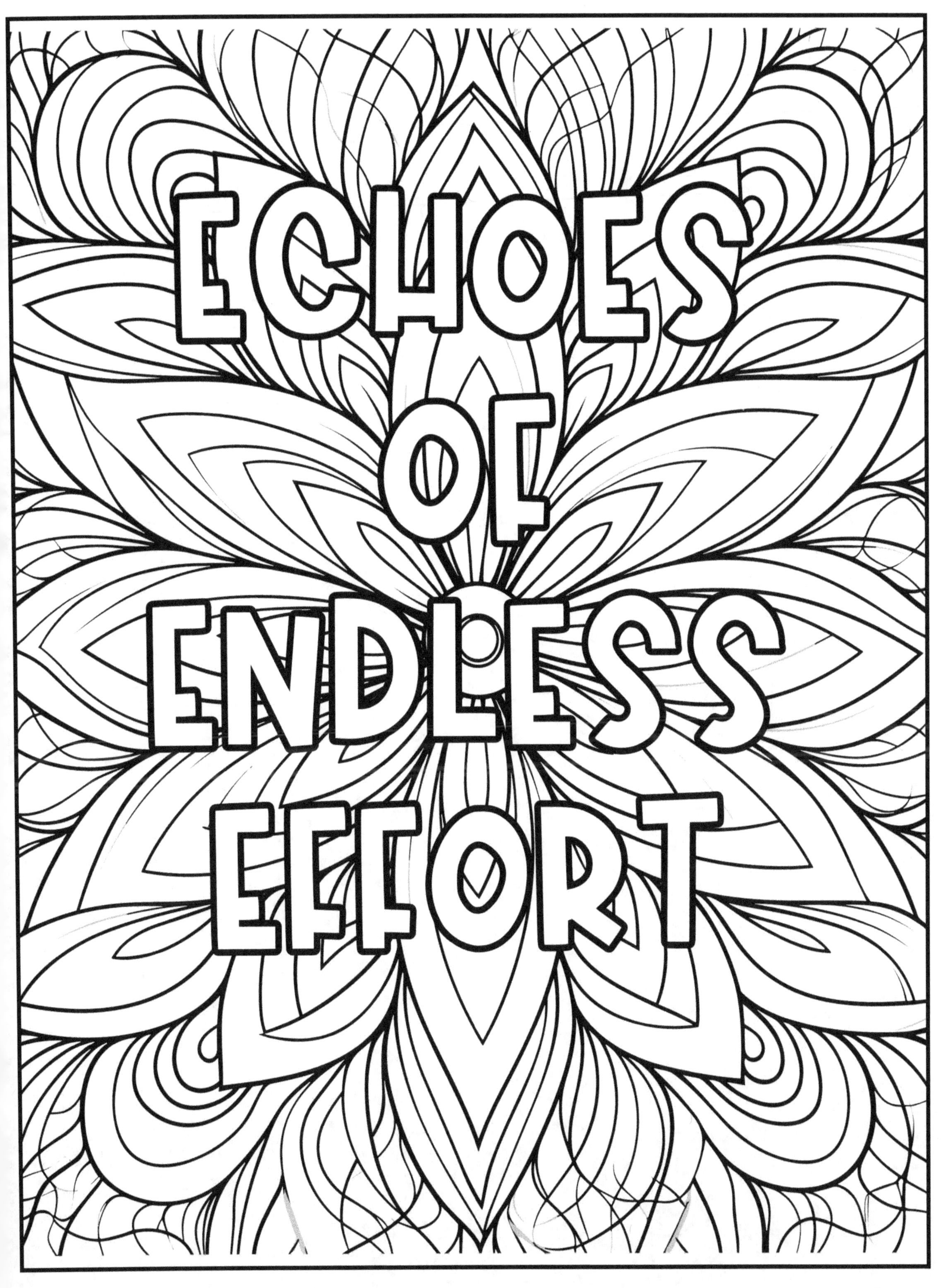

ECHOES
OF
ENDLESS
EFFORT

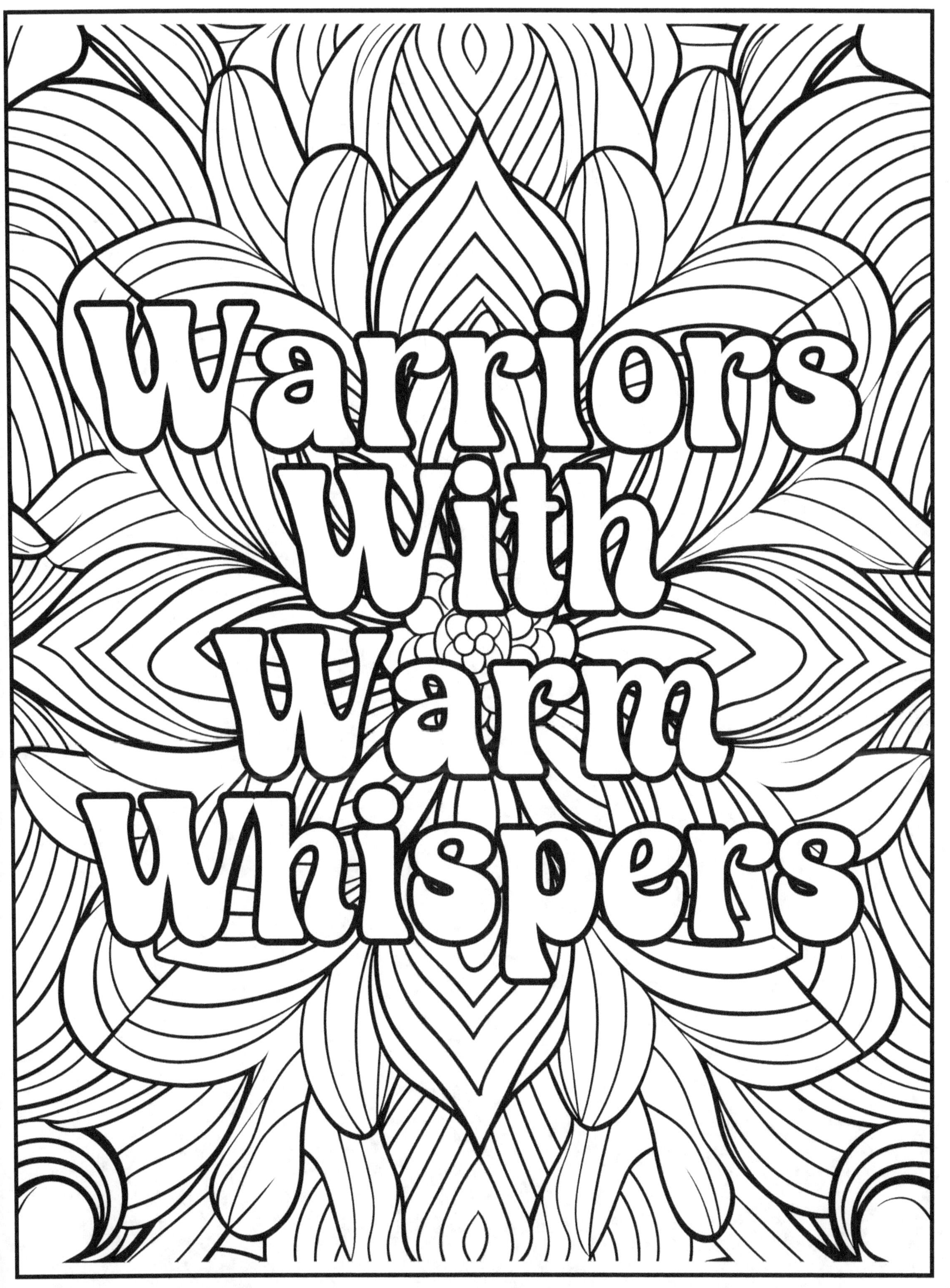

Warriors
With
Warm
Whispers

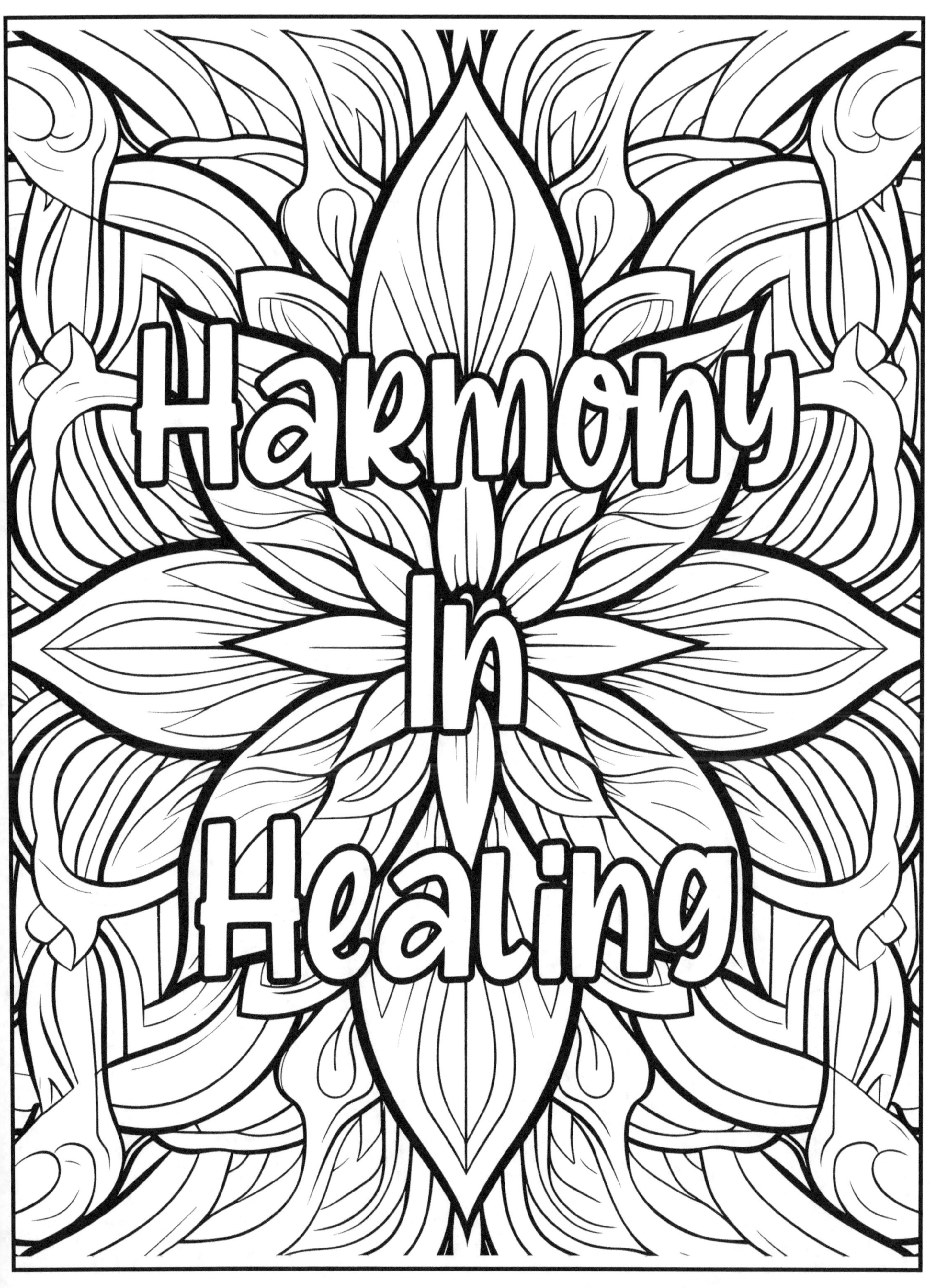

Harmony
In
Healing

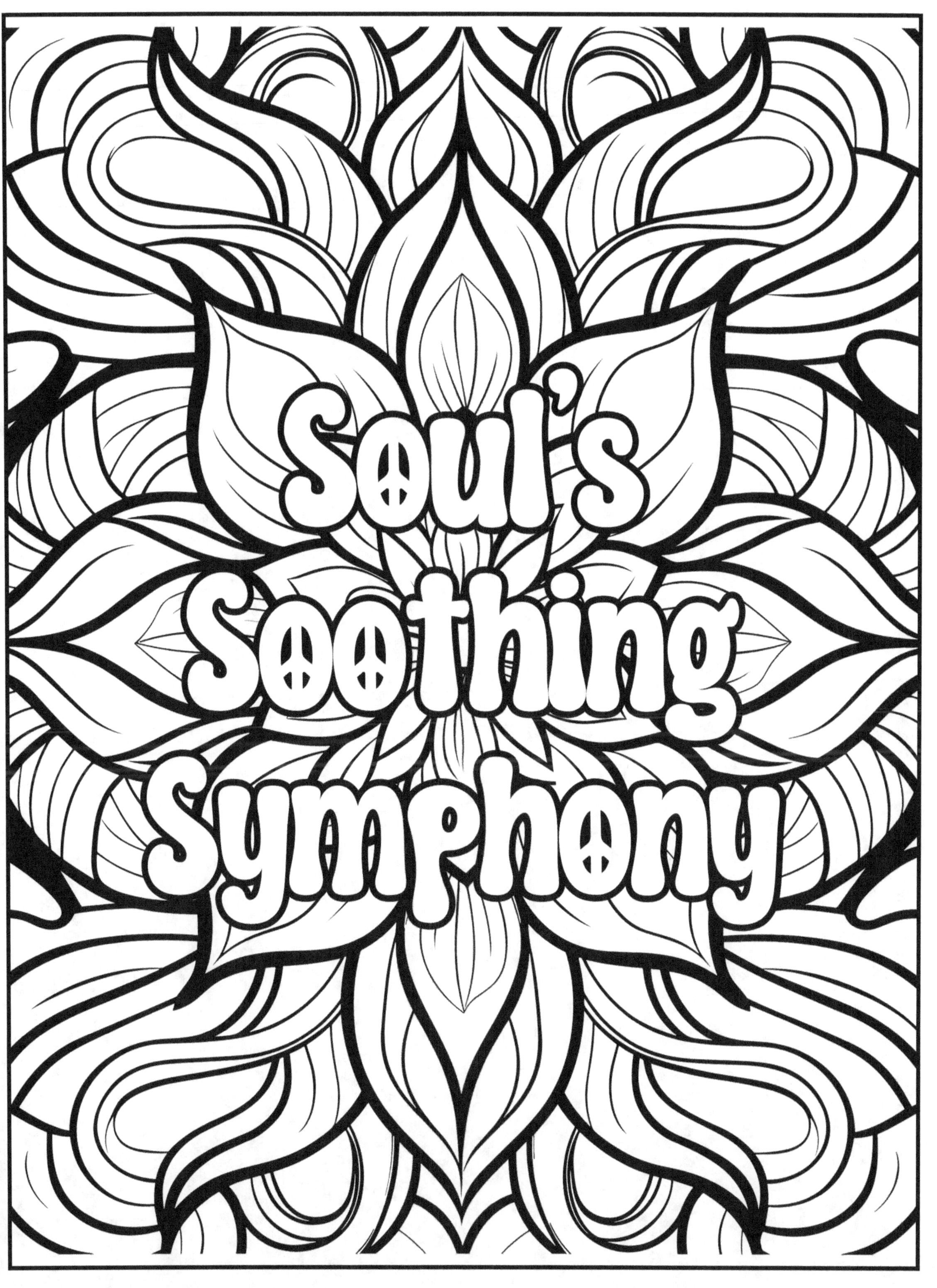

Soul's
Soothing
Symphony

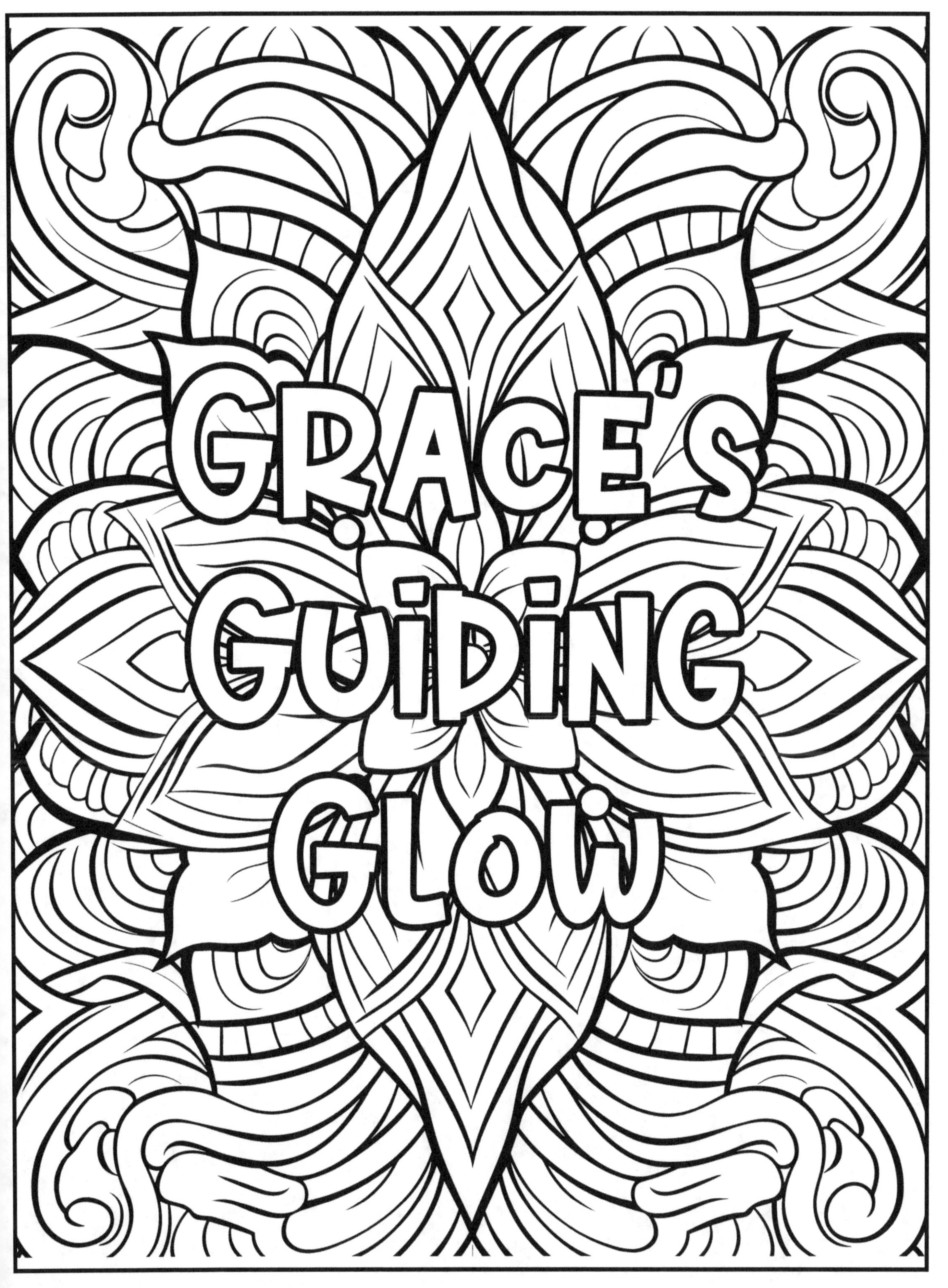

Grace's
Guiding
Glow

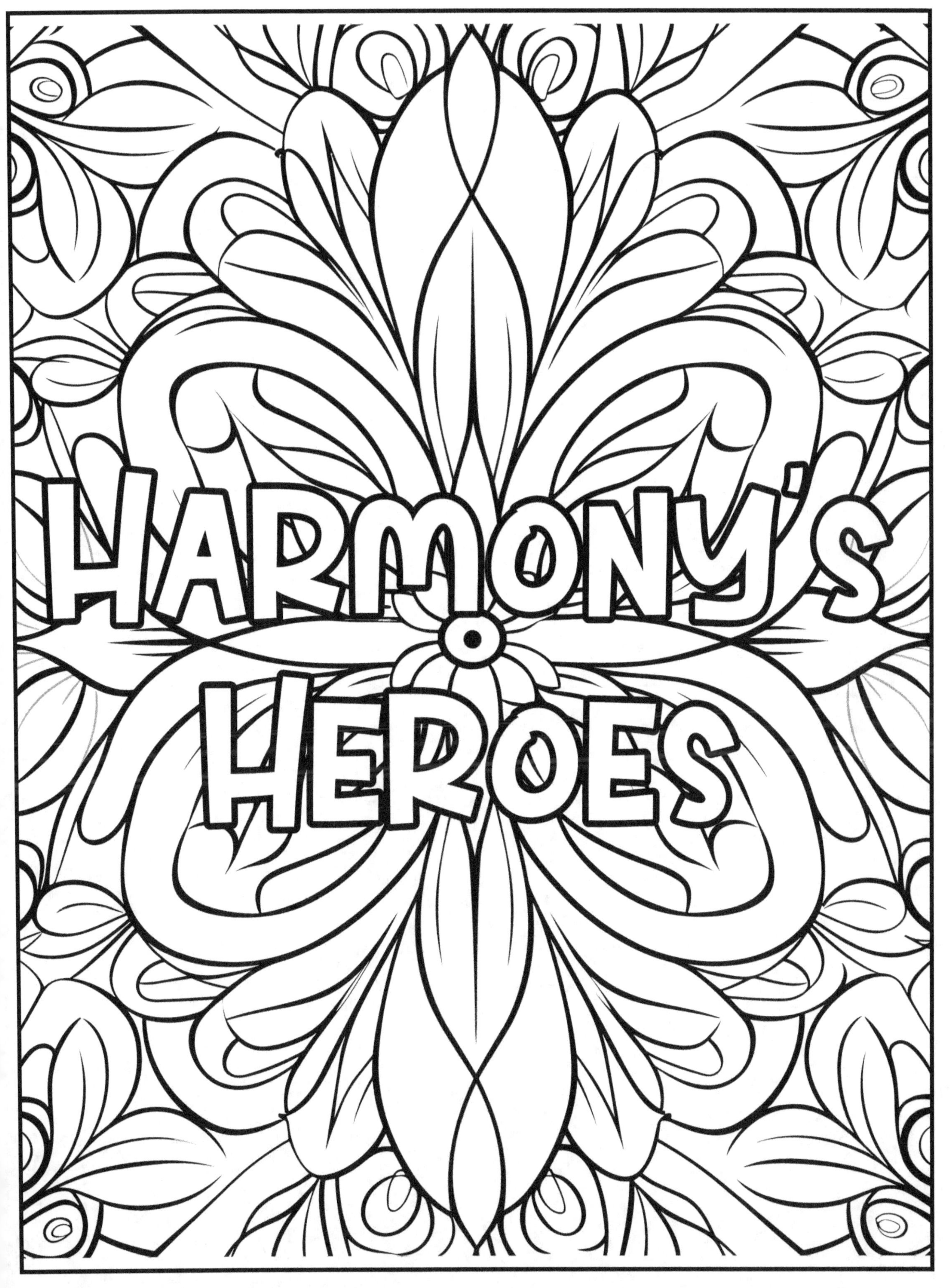

HARMONY'S
HEROES

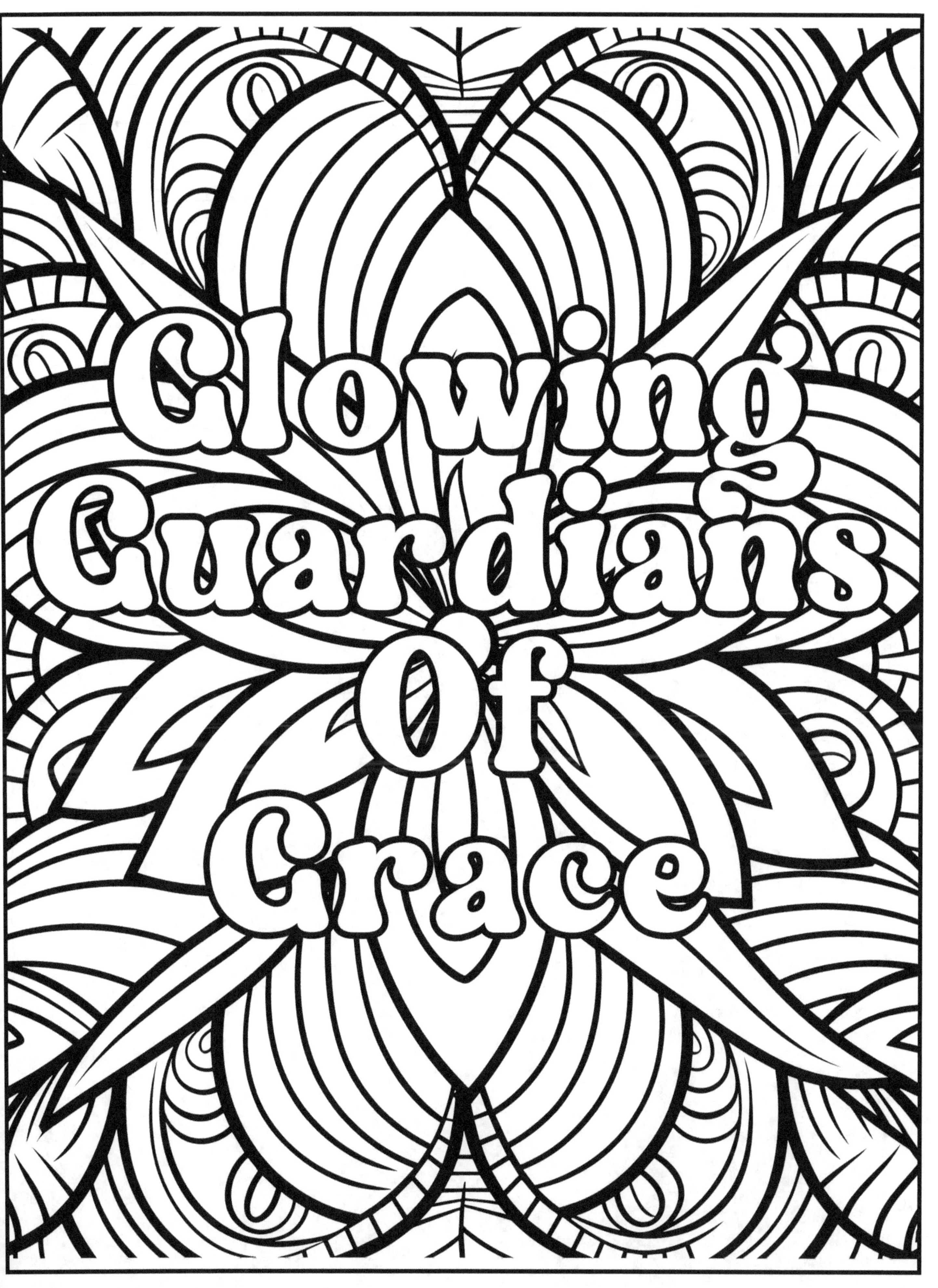

Glowing
Guardians
Of
Grace

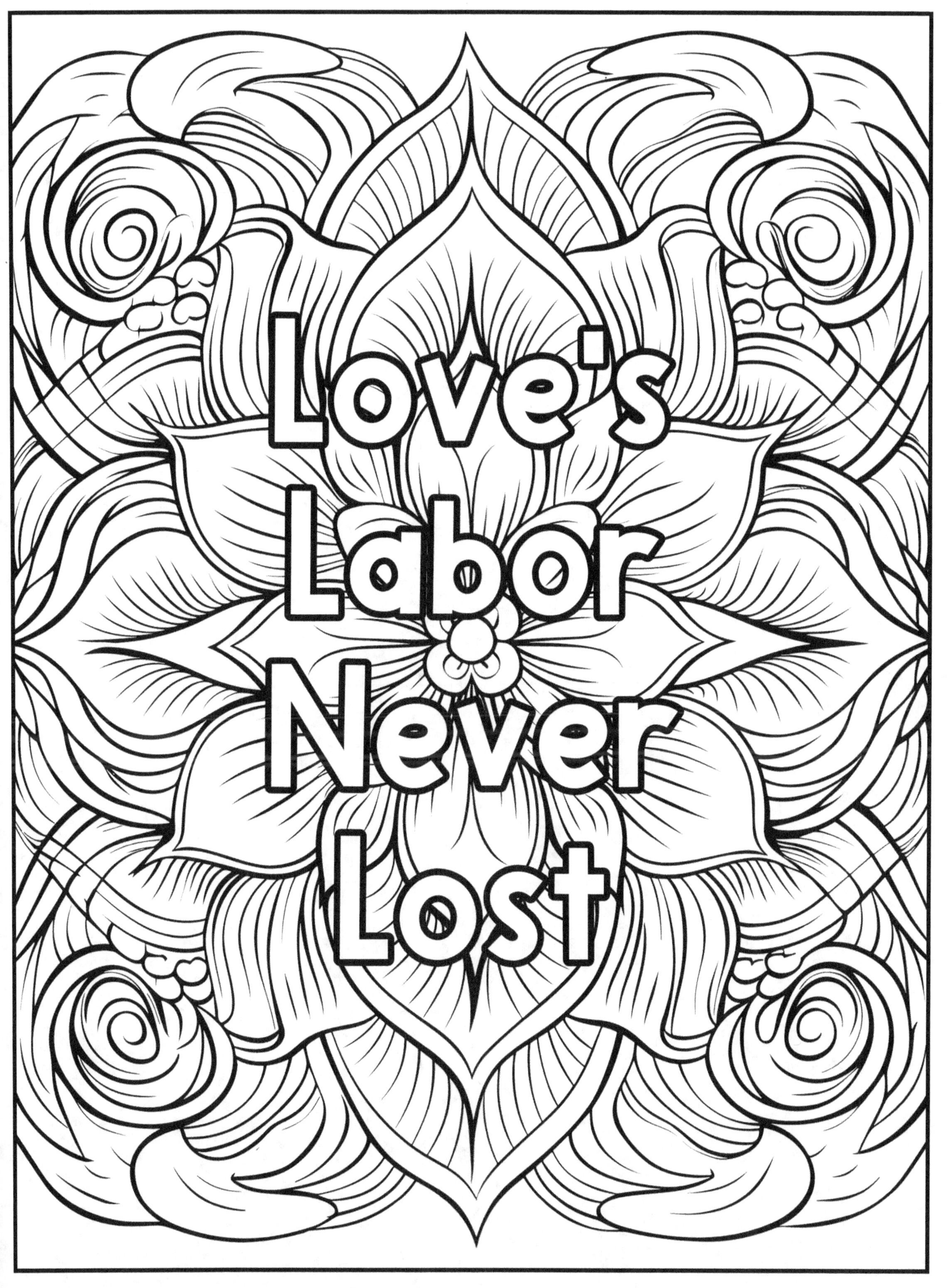

Love's
Labor
Never
Lost

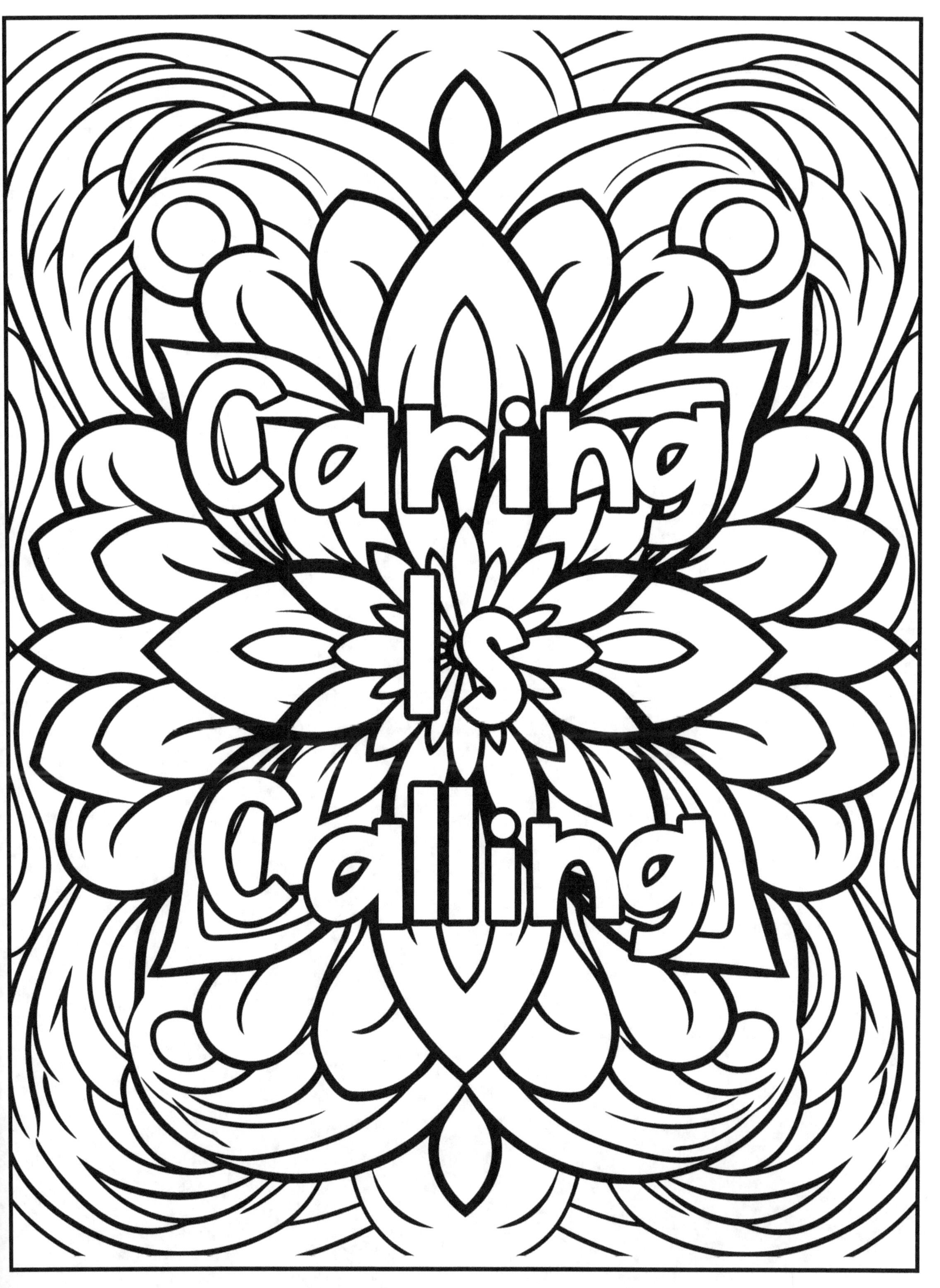

Caring
Is
Calling

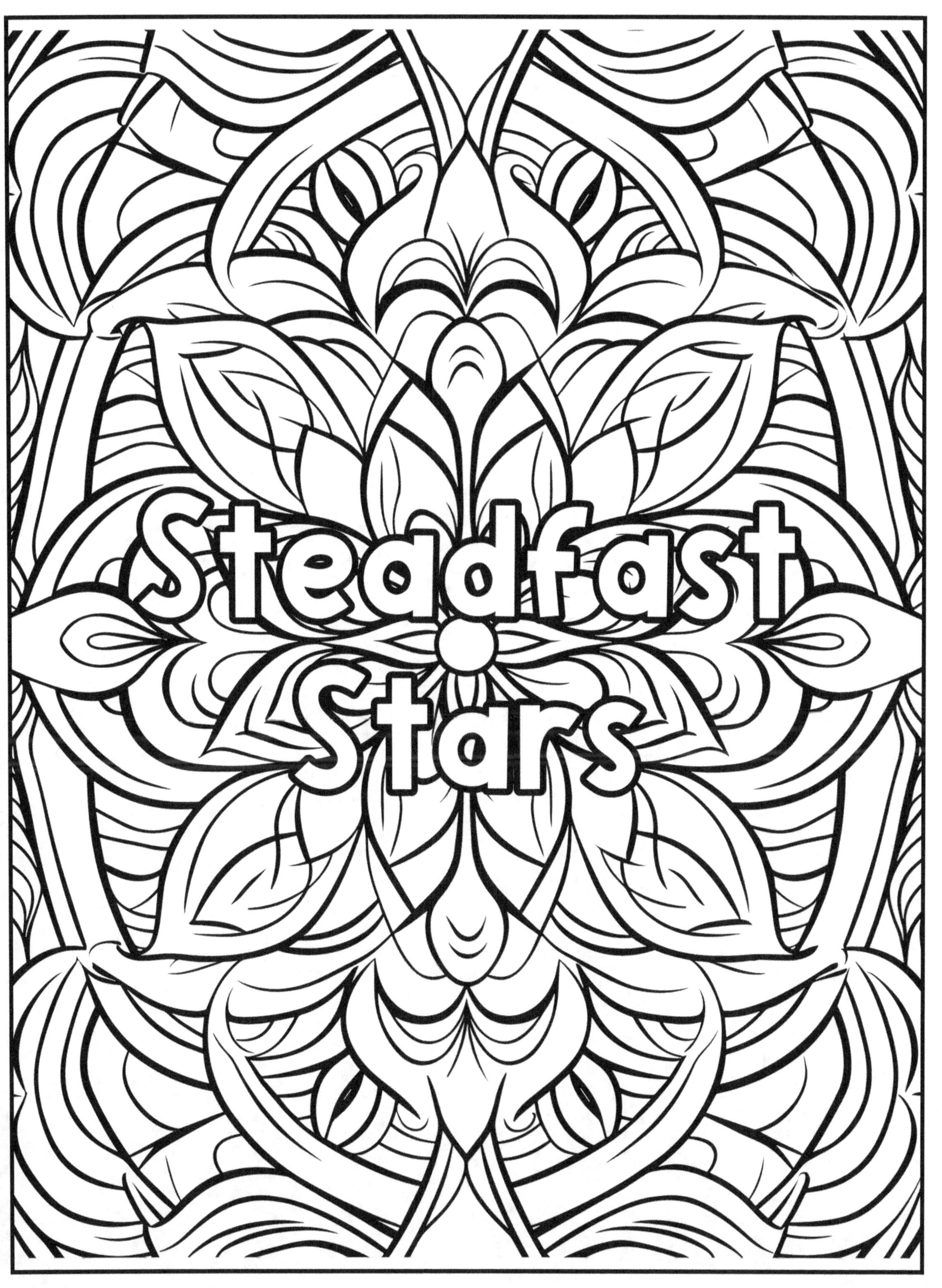
Steadfast
Stars

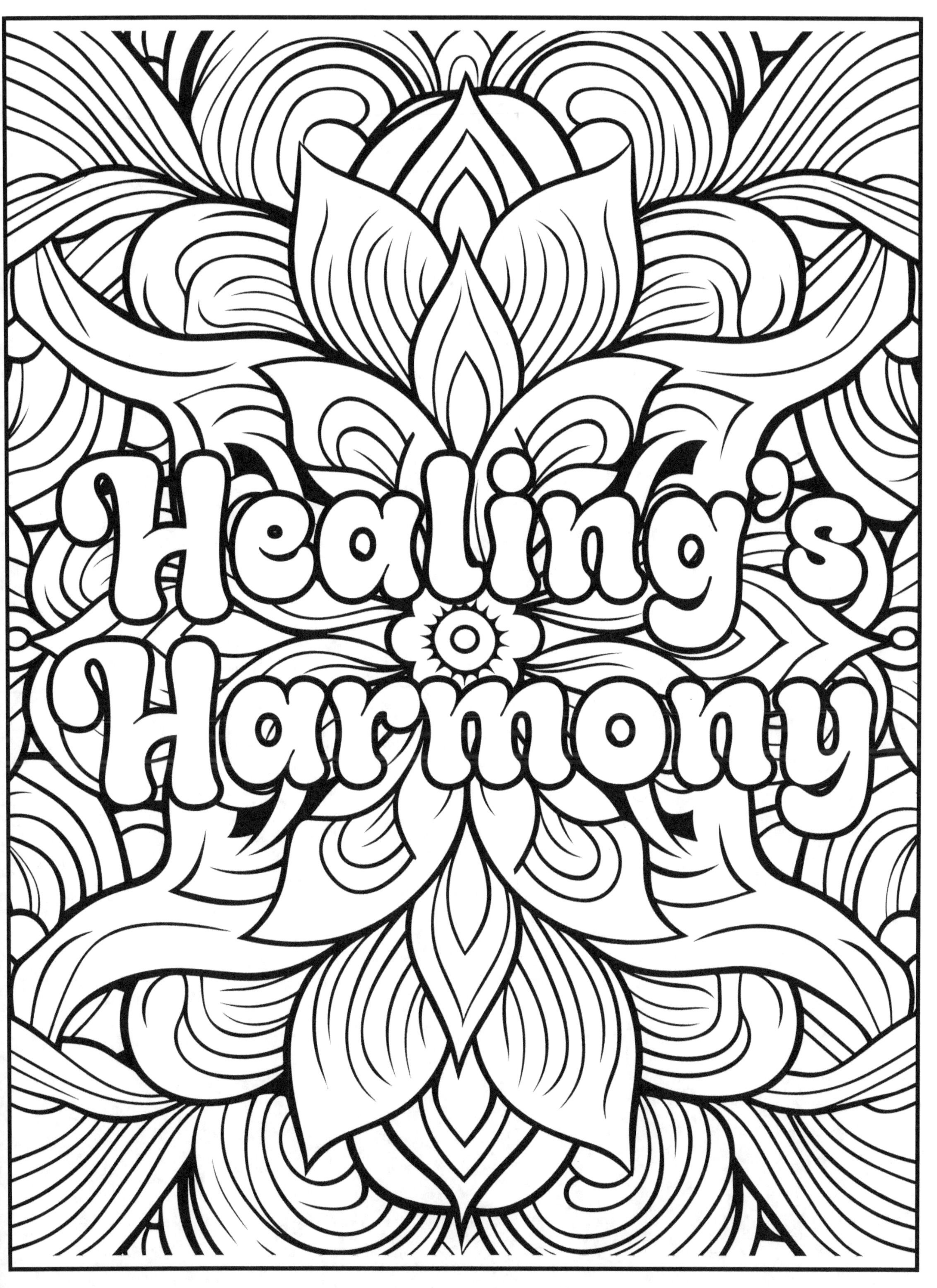

Healing's
Harmony

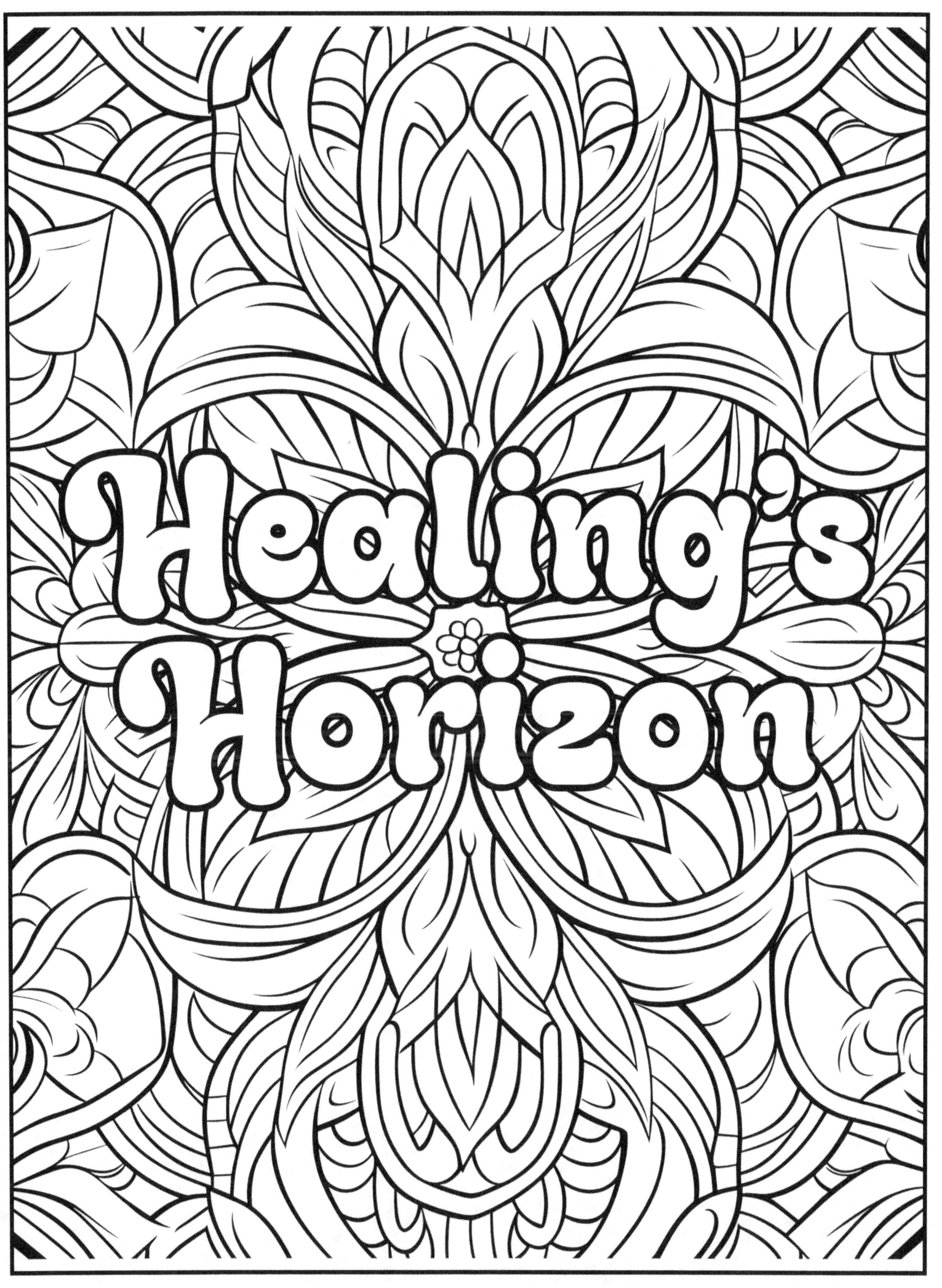

Healing's
Horizon

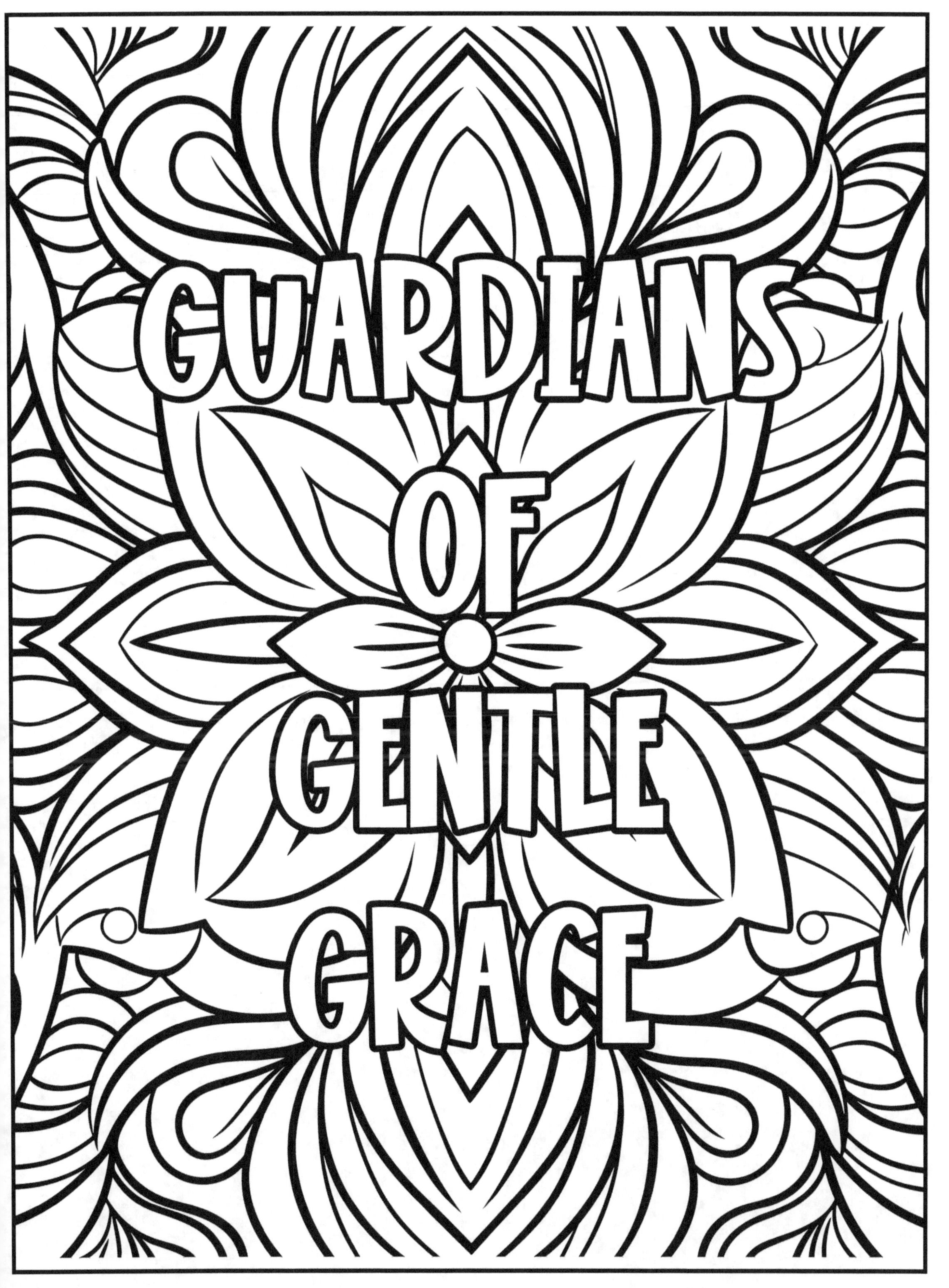

GUARDIANS
OF
GENTLE
GRACE

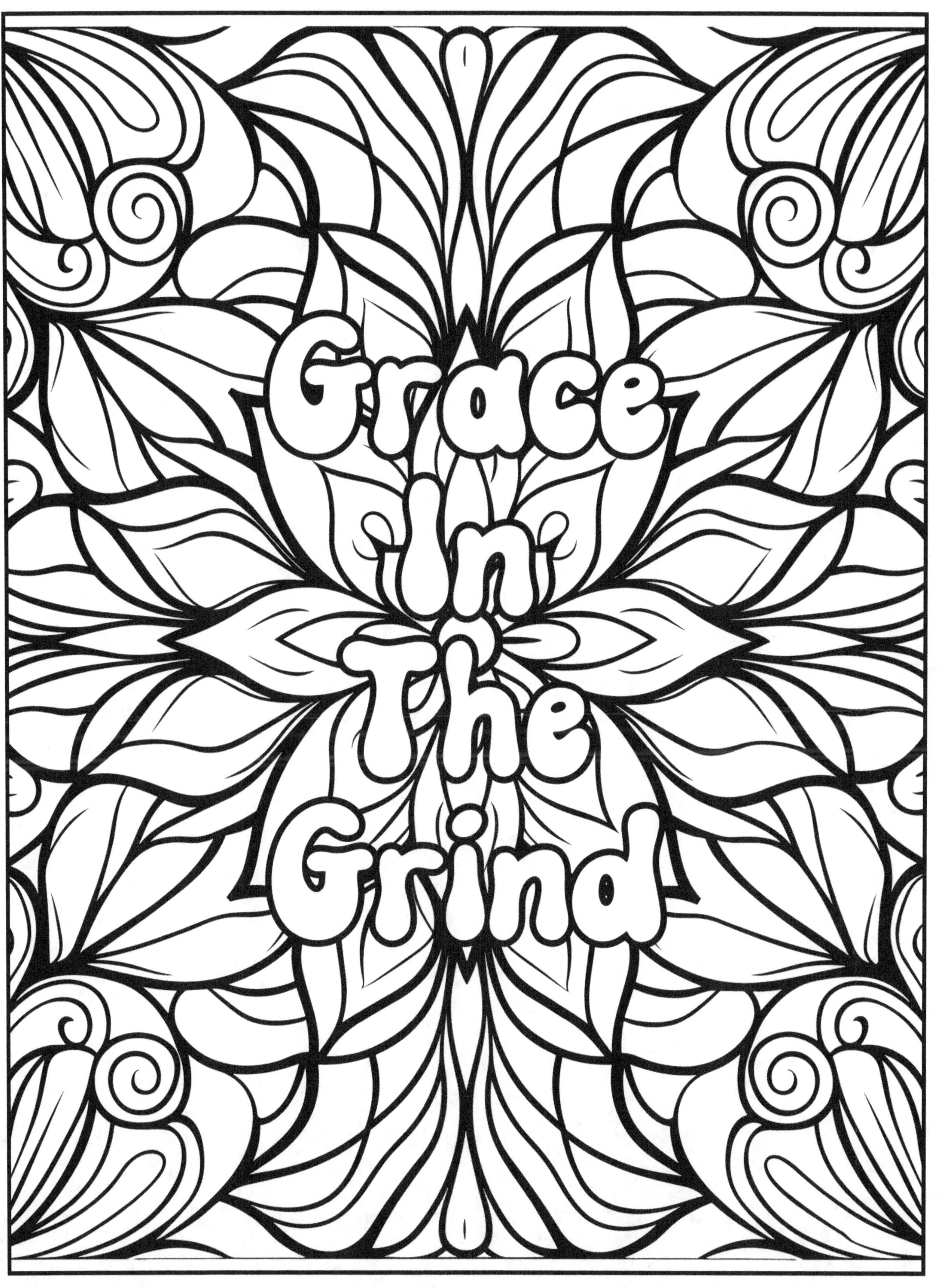

Grace
In
The
Grind

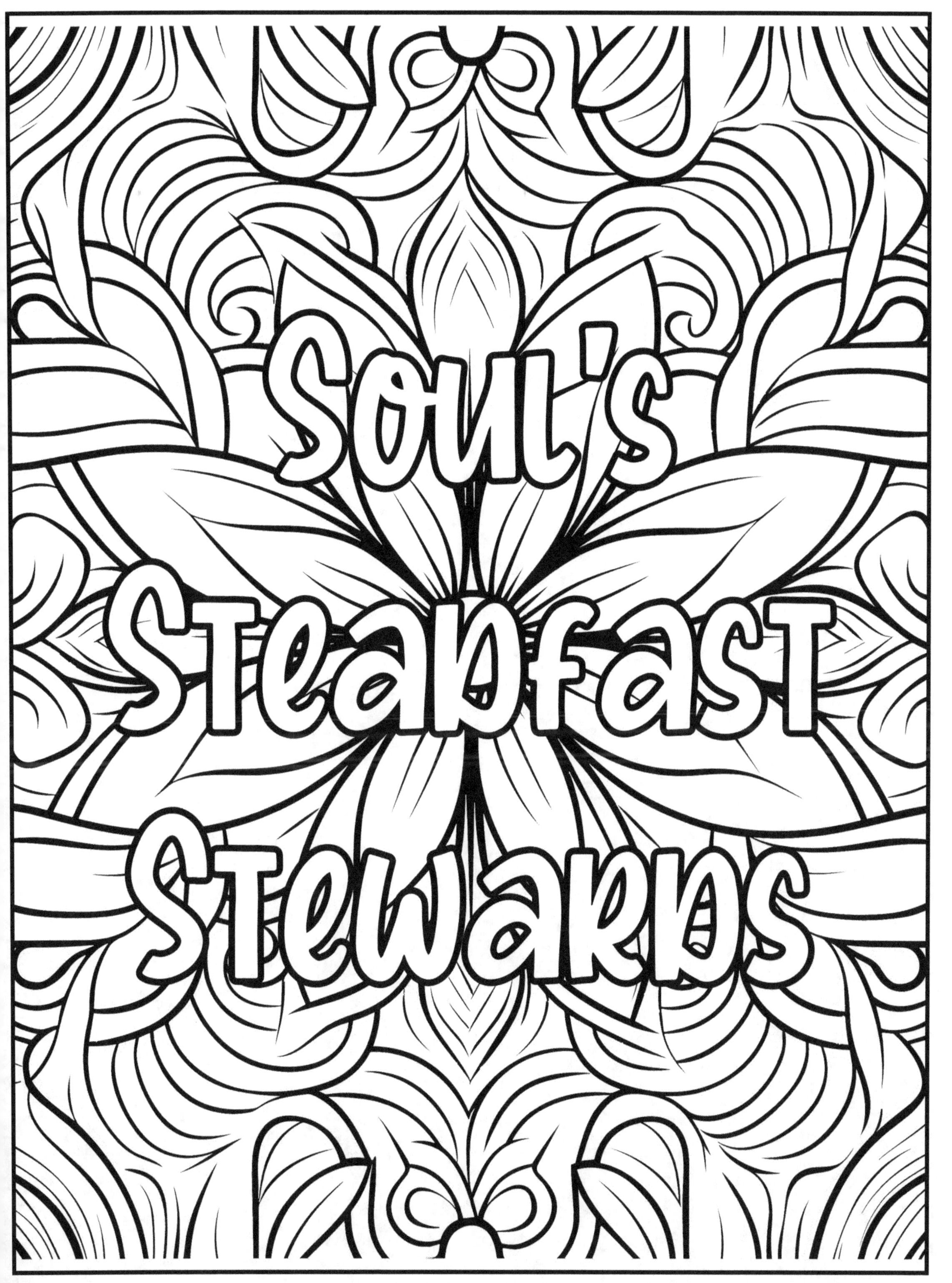
Soul's
Steadfast
Stewards

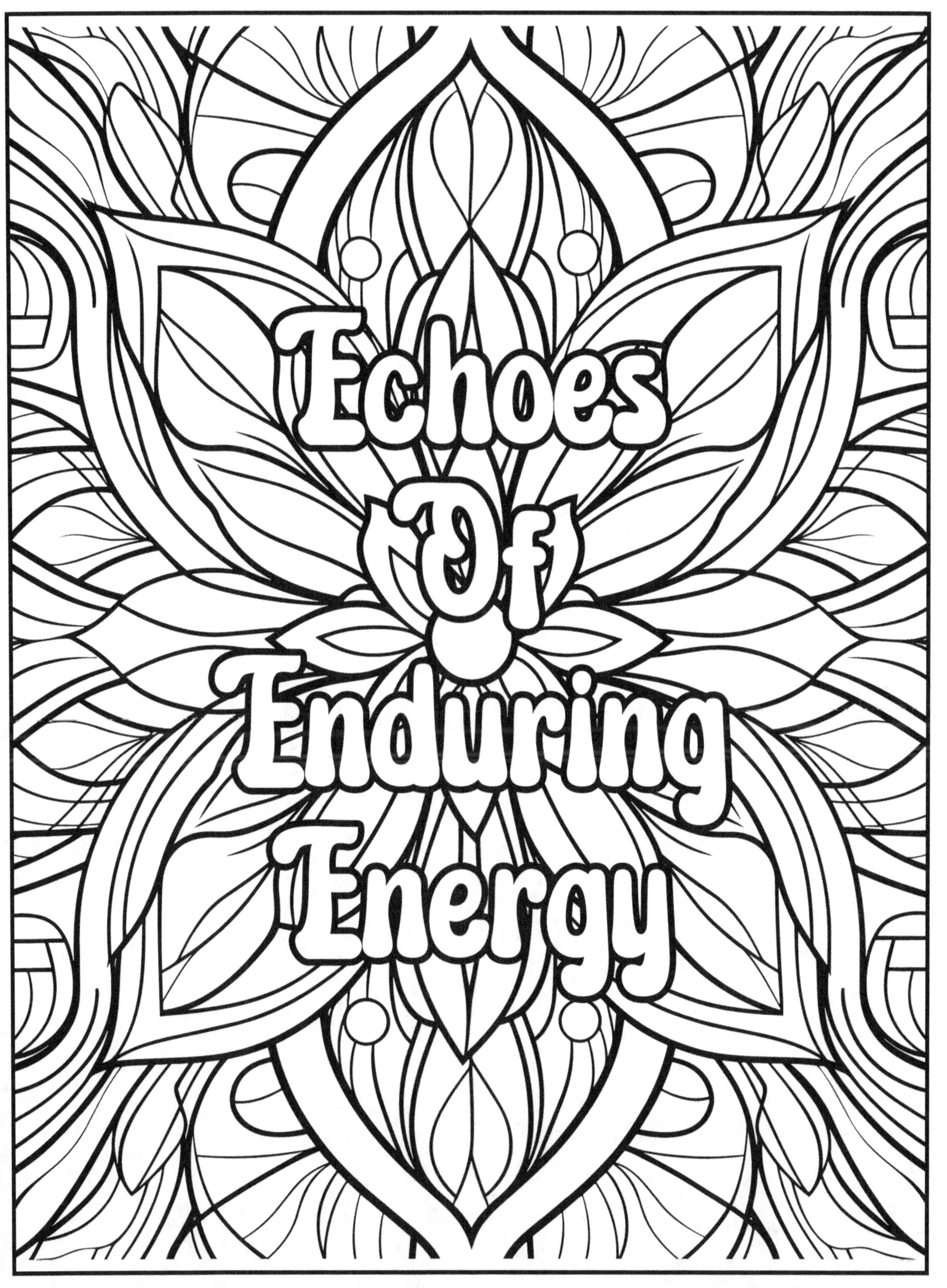
Echoes
Of
Enduring
Energy

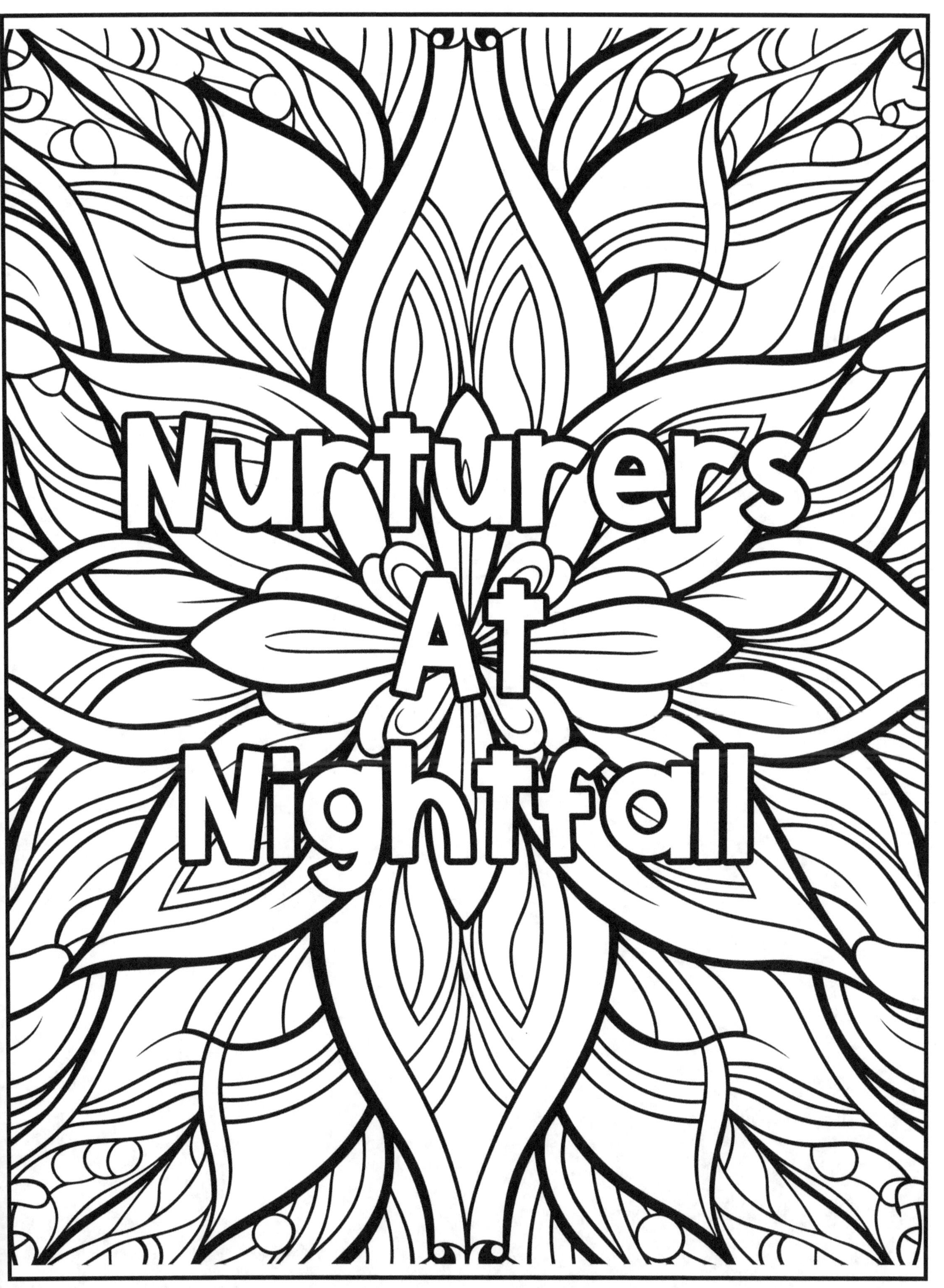

Nurturers
At
Nightfall

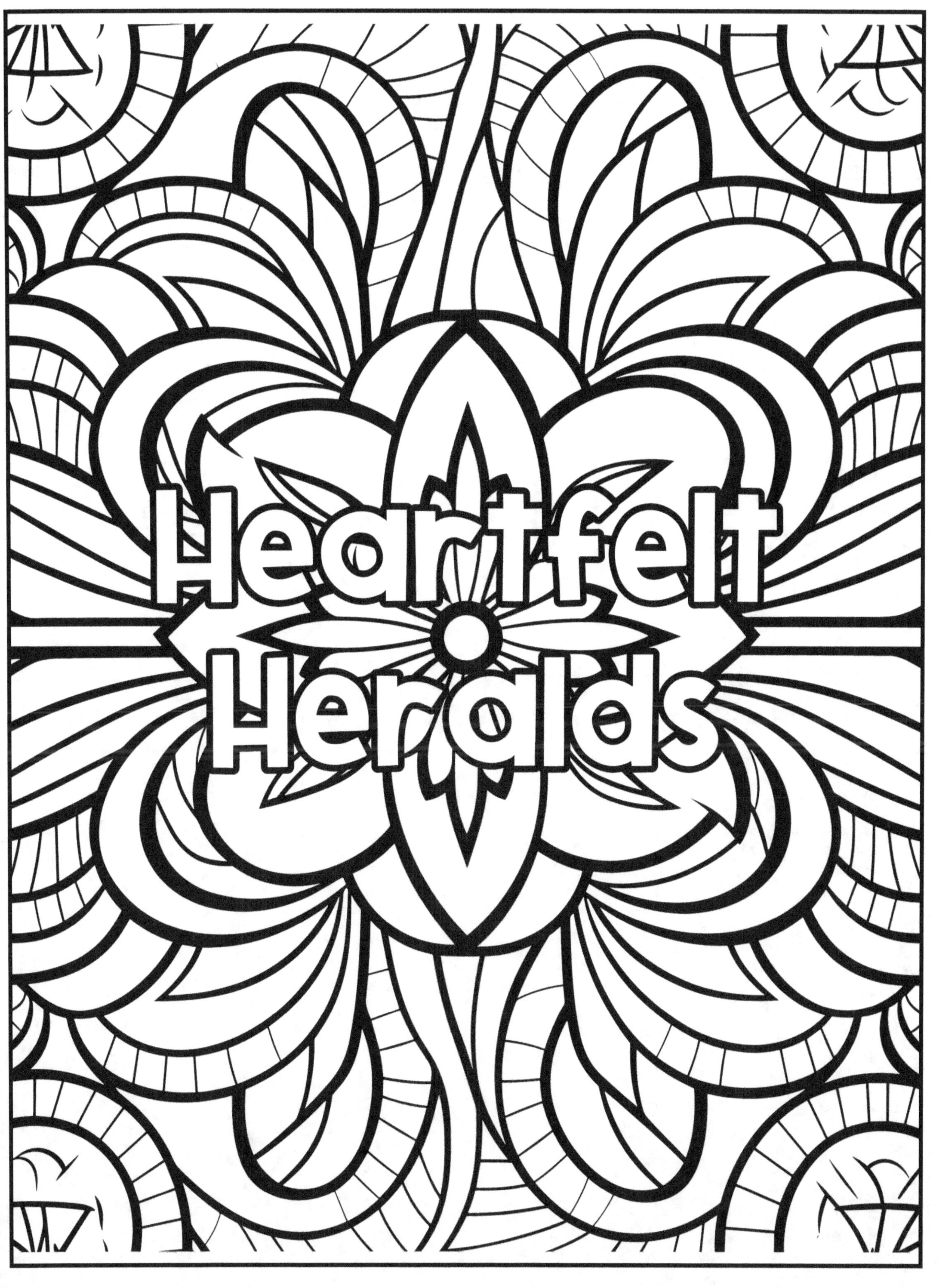

Heartfelt
Heralds

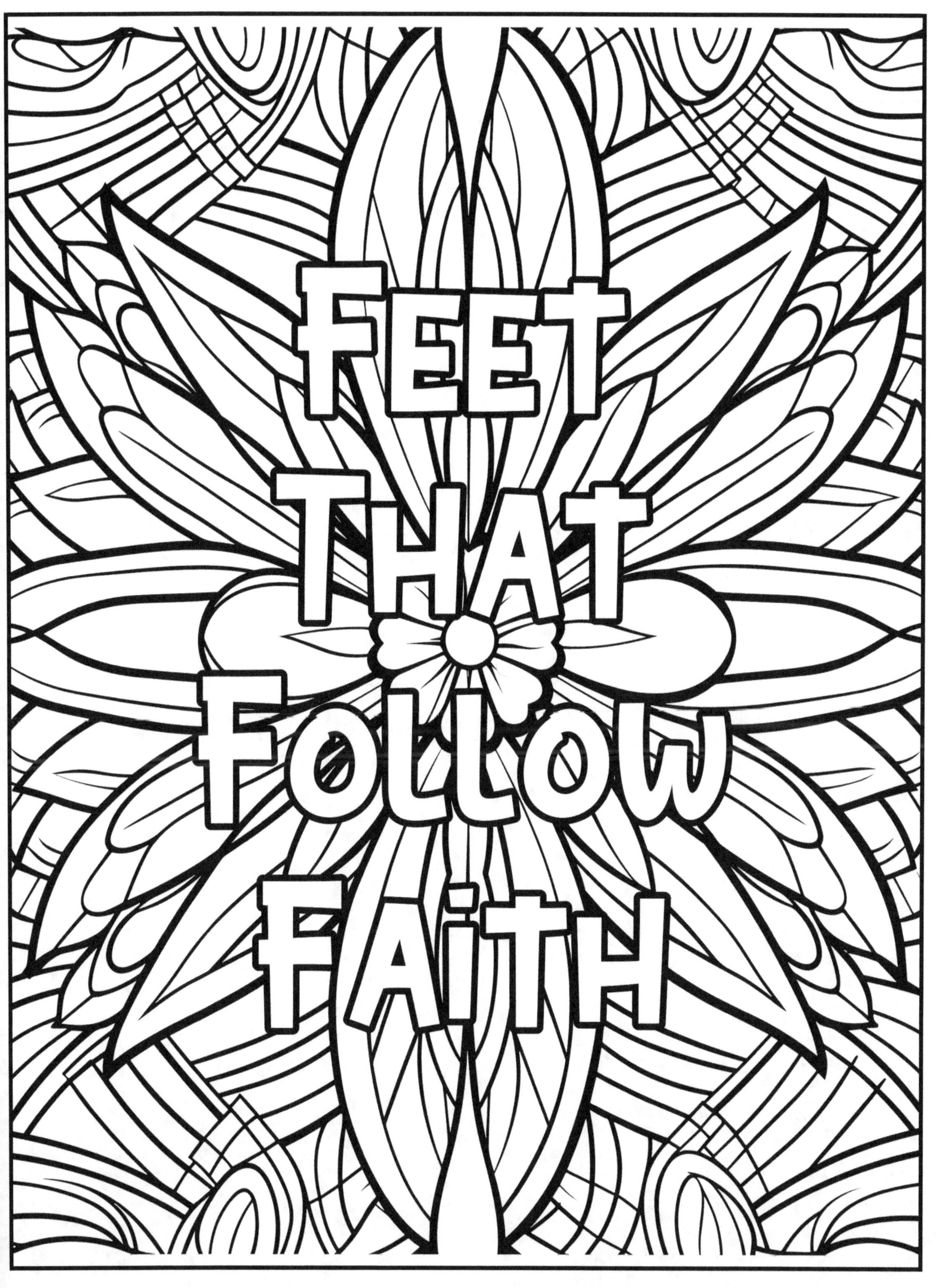
FEET
THAT
FOLLOW
FAITH

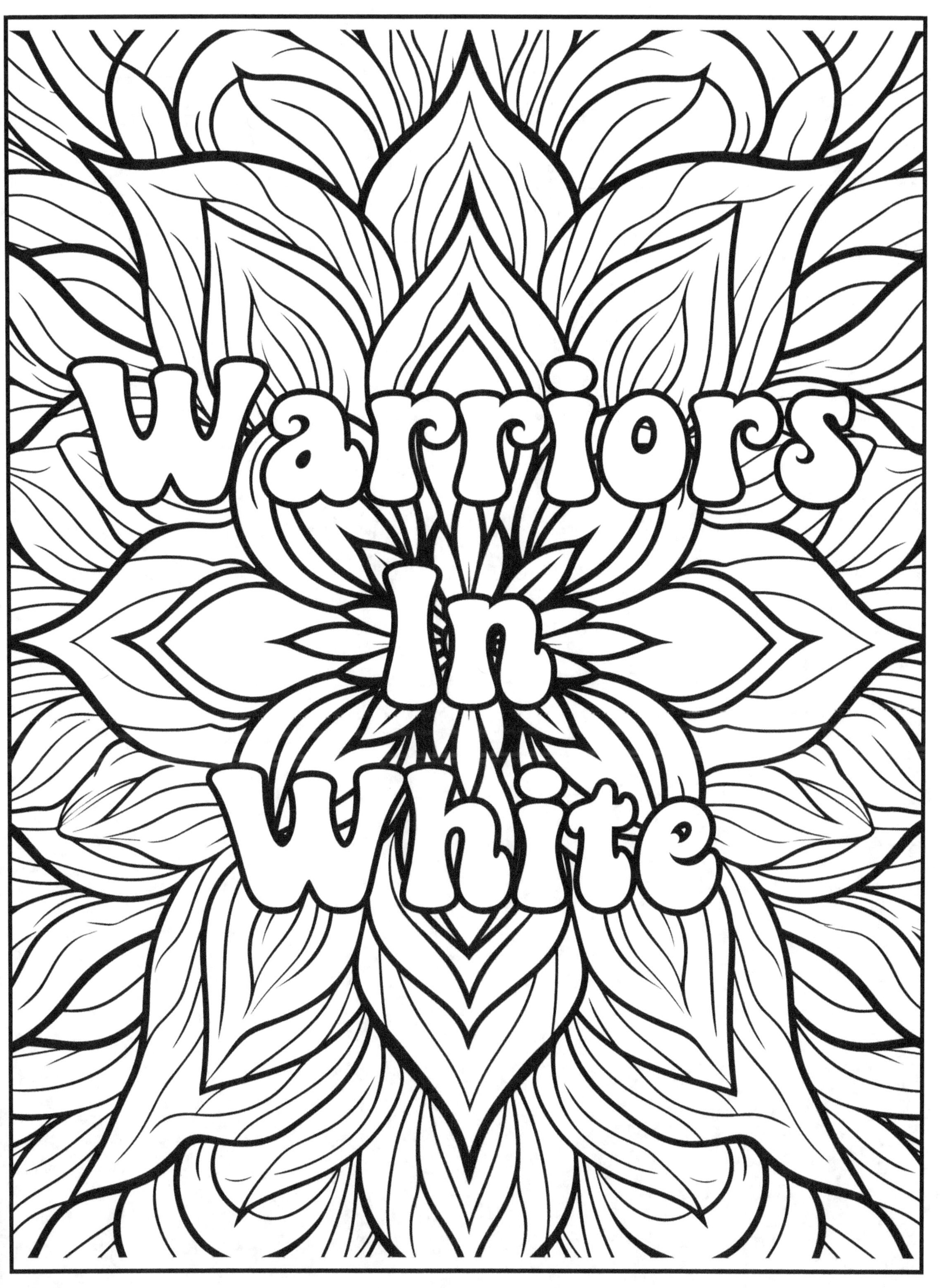

Warriors
In
White

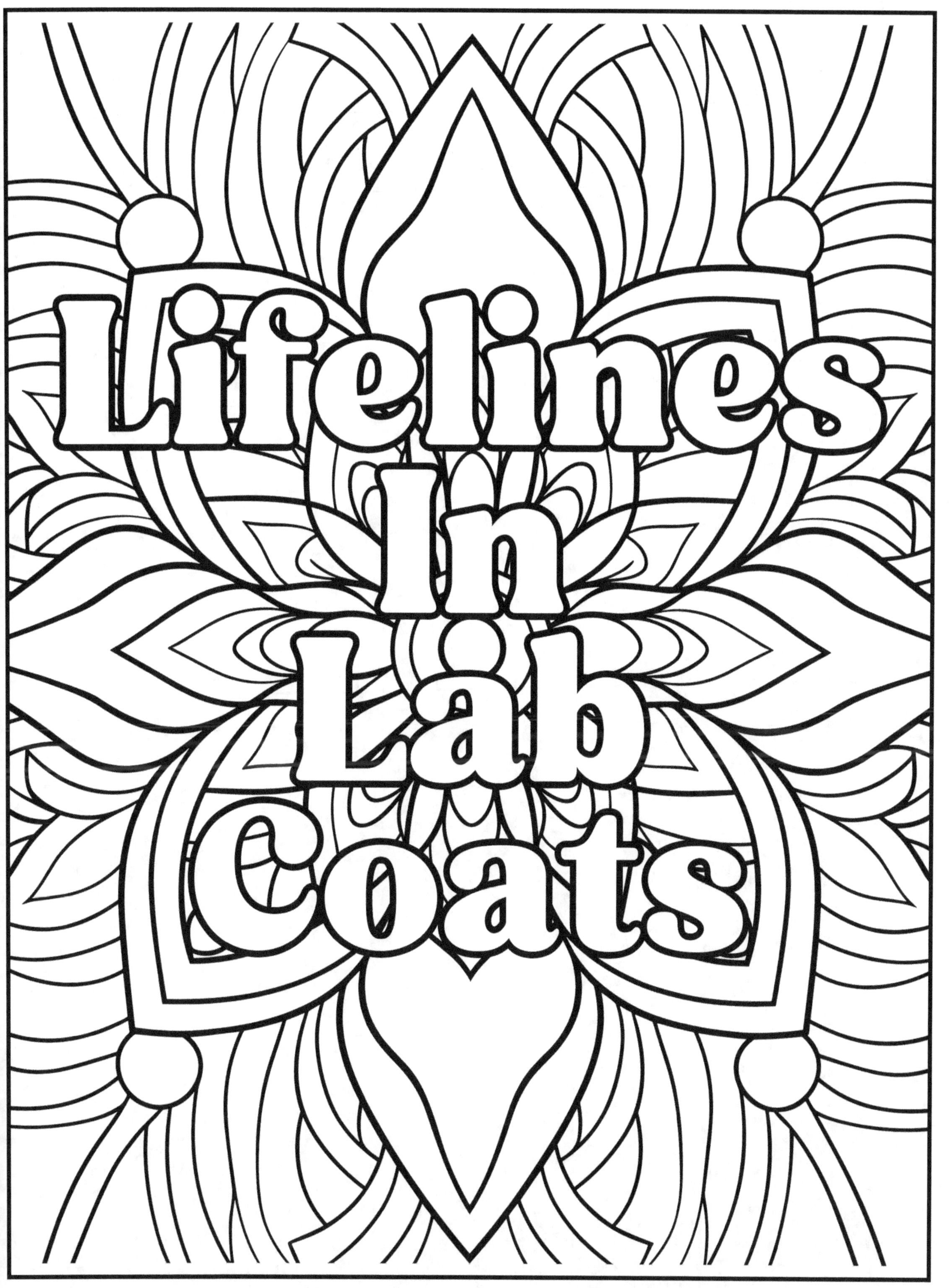

Lifelines
In
Lab
Coats

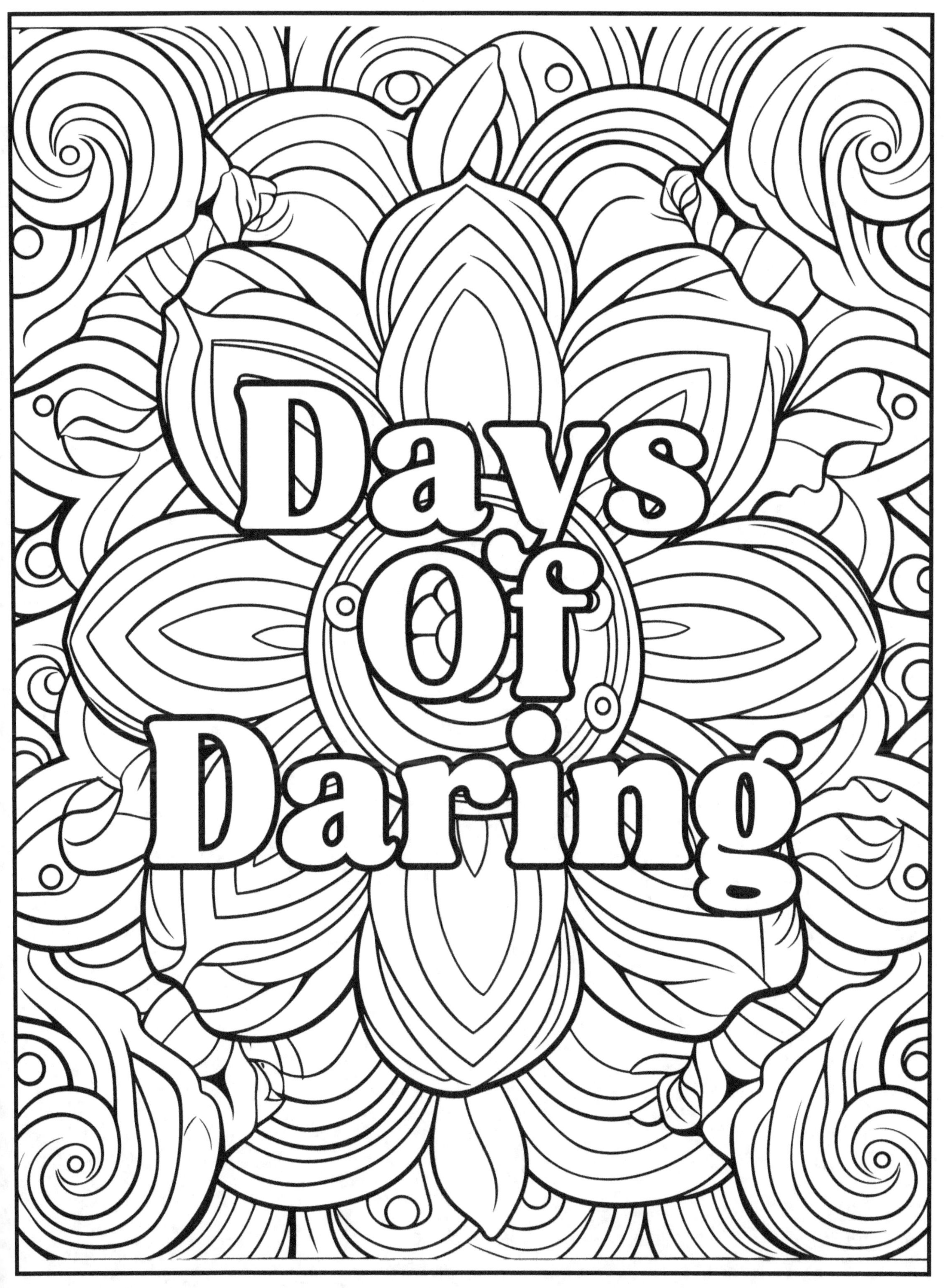

Days
Of
Daring

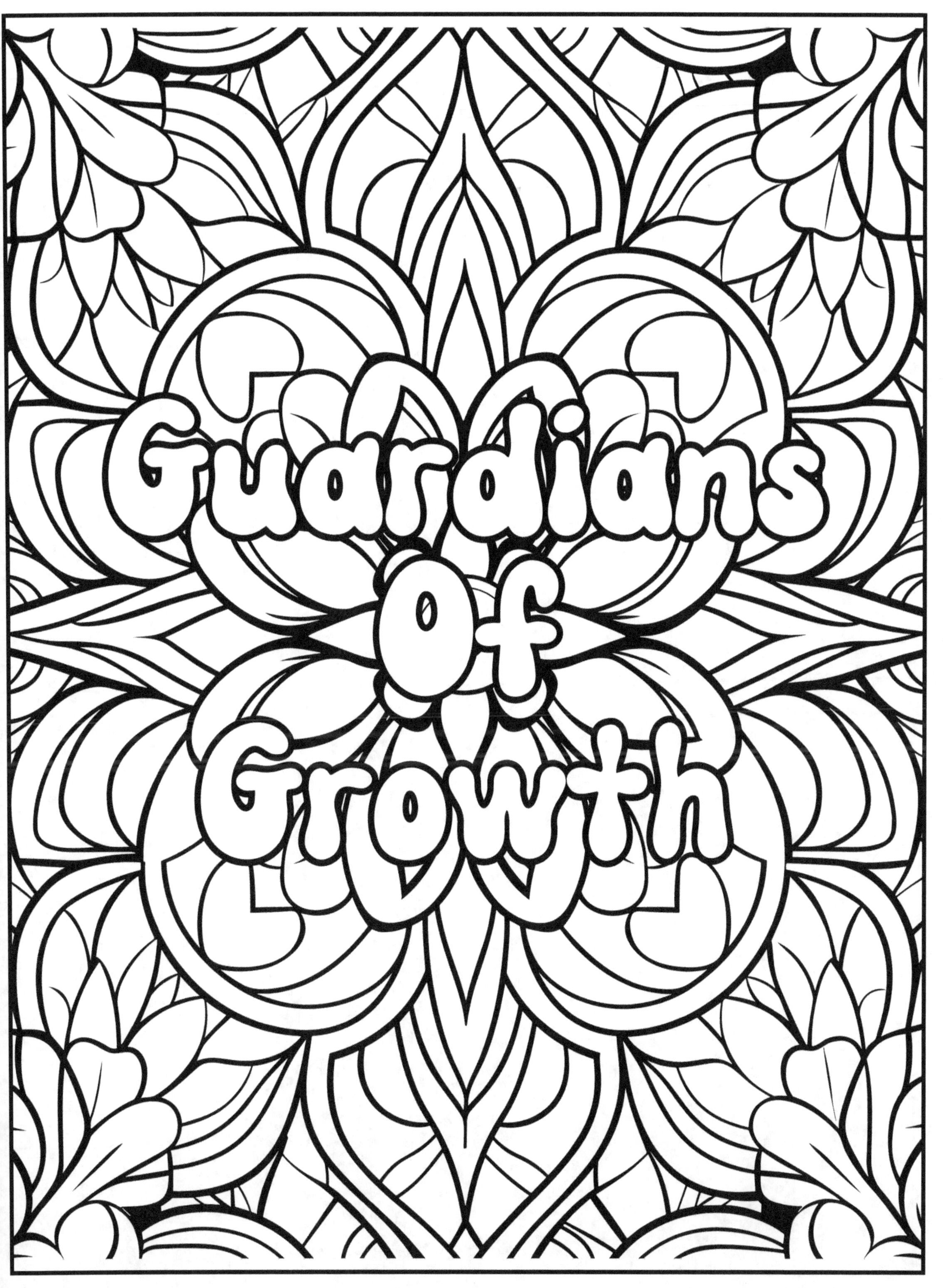

Guardians
Of
Growth

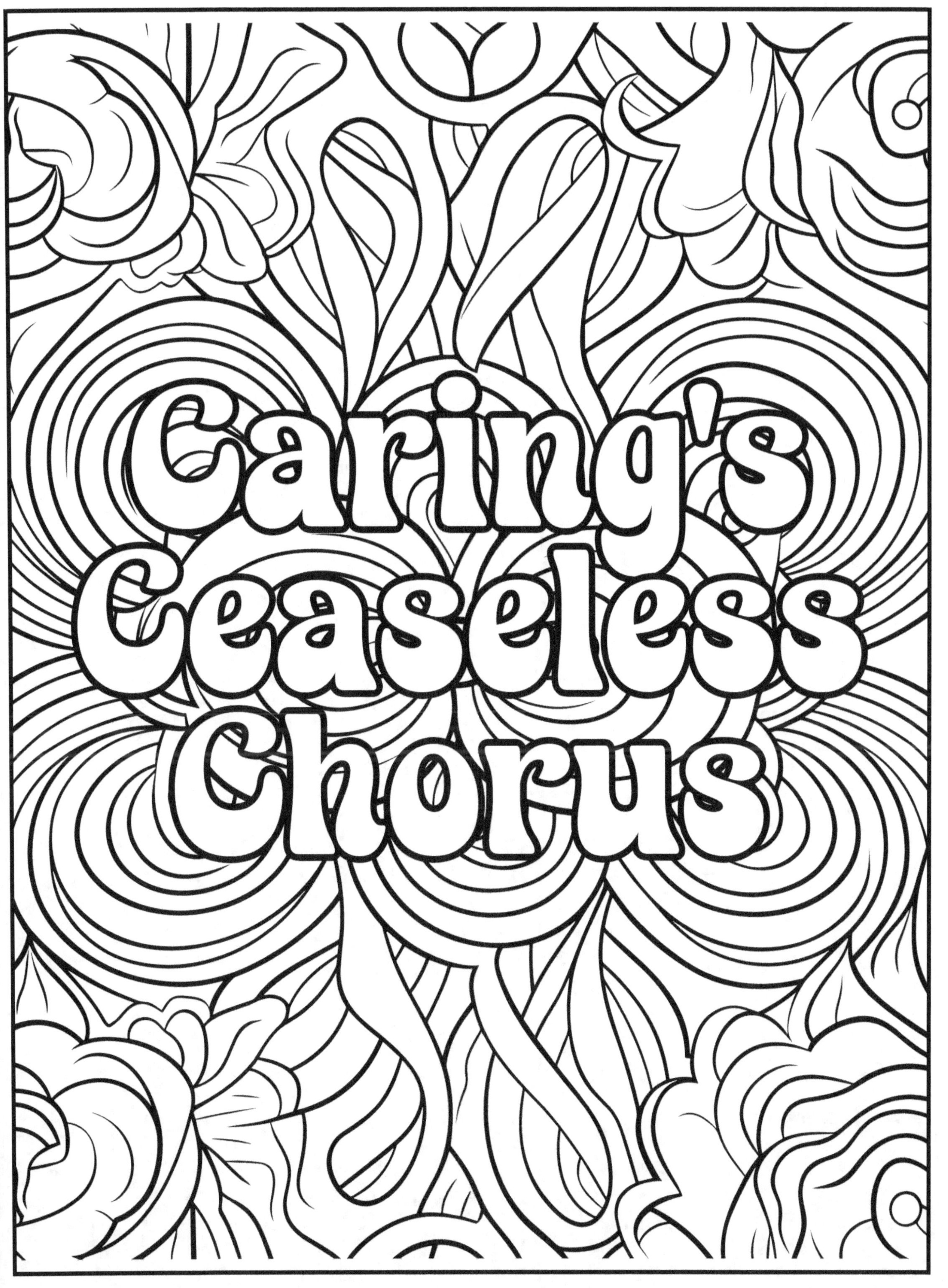

Caring's
Ceaseless
Chorus

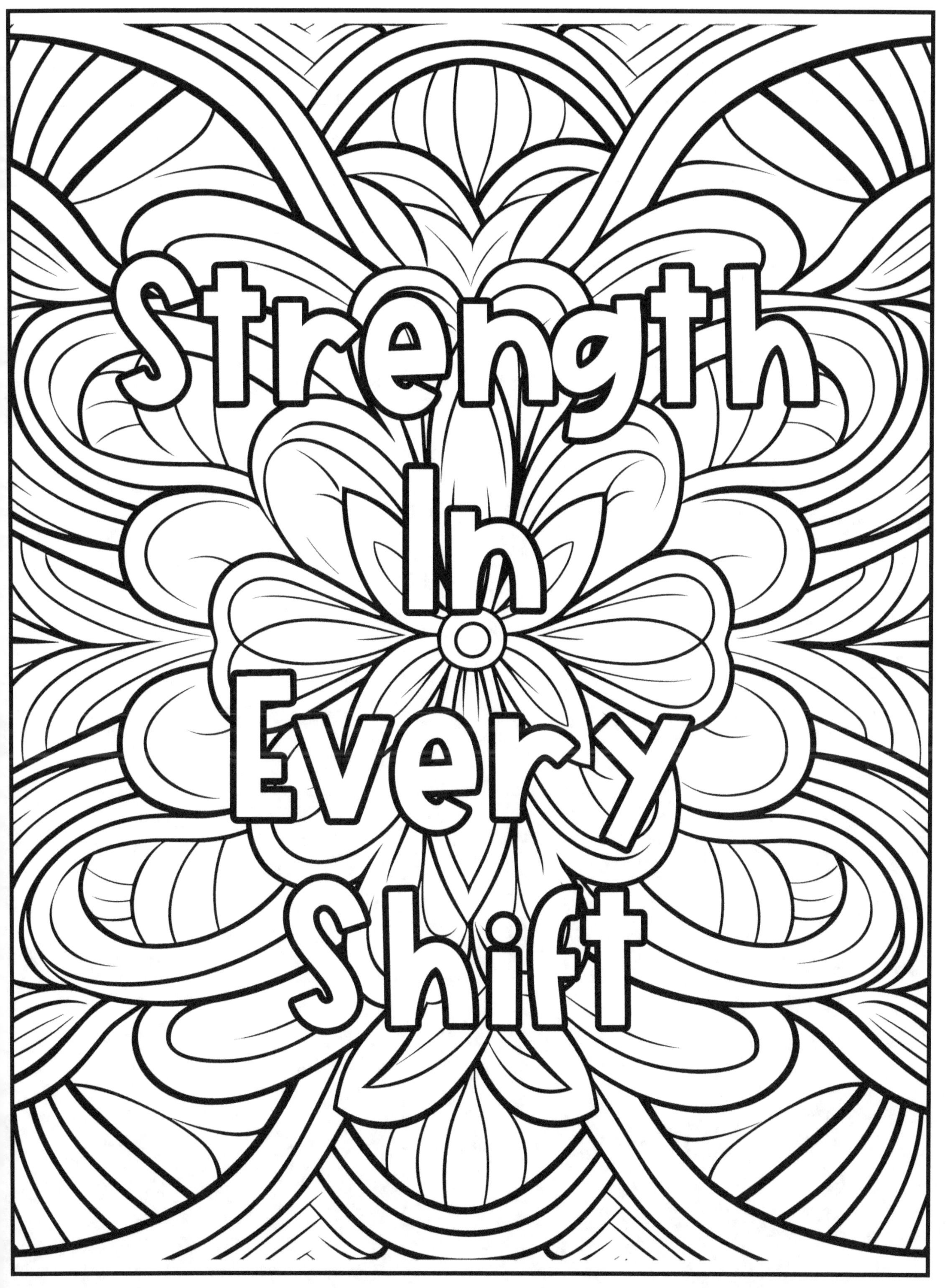

Strength
In
Every
Shift

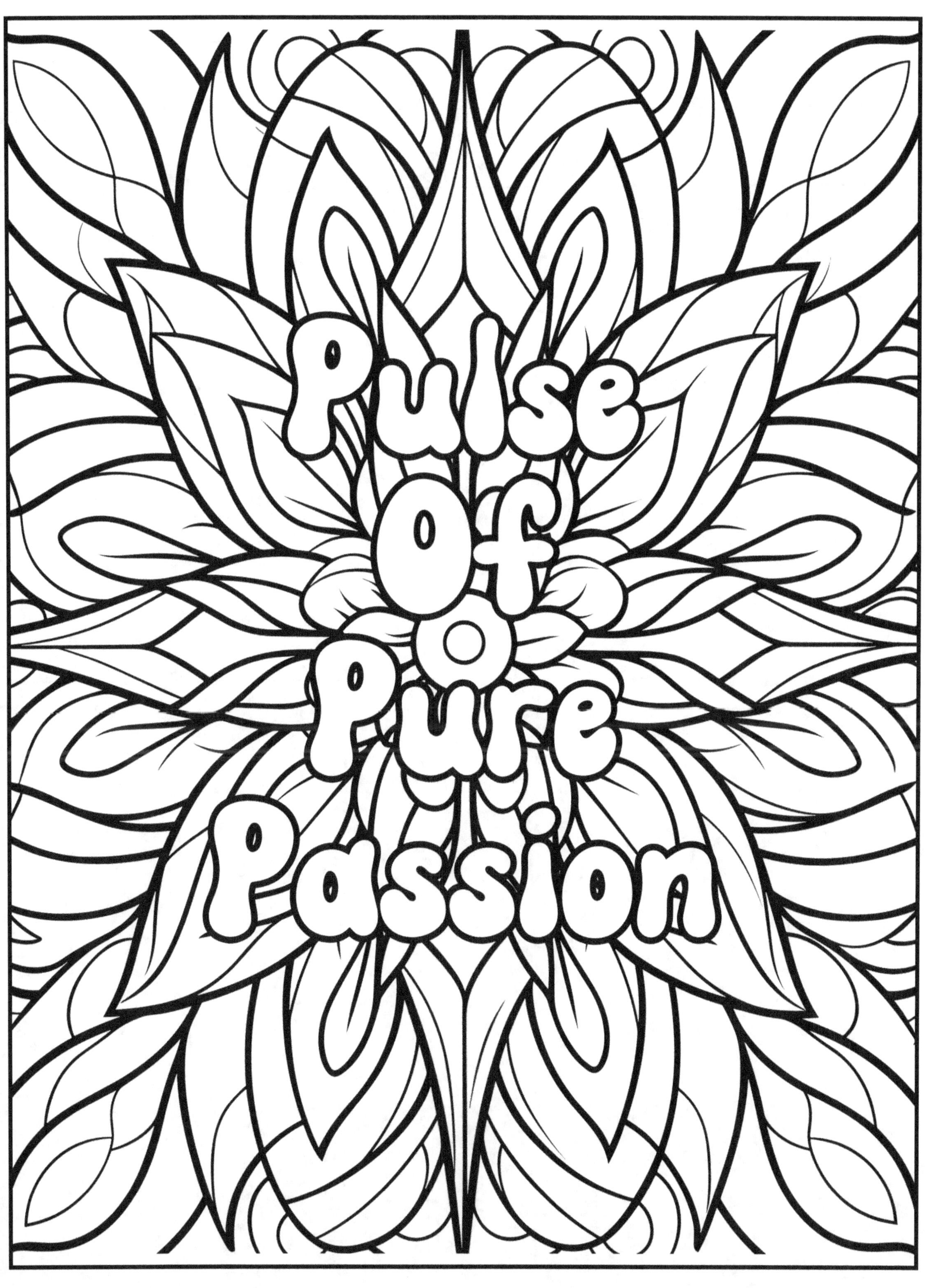

Pulse
Of
O
Pure
Passion

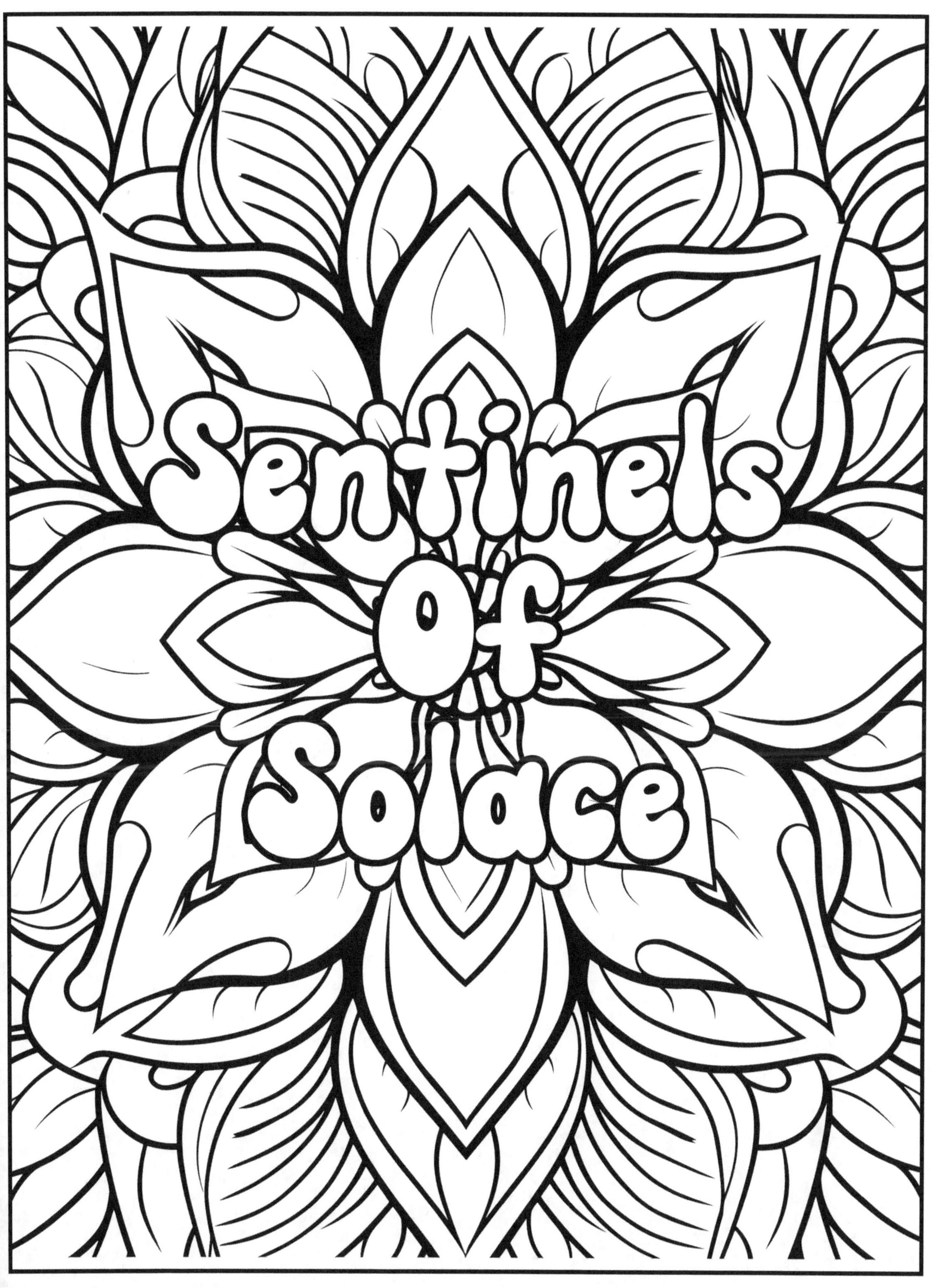

Sentinels
Of
Solace

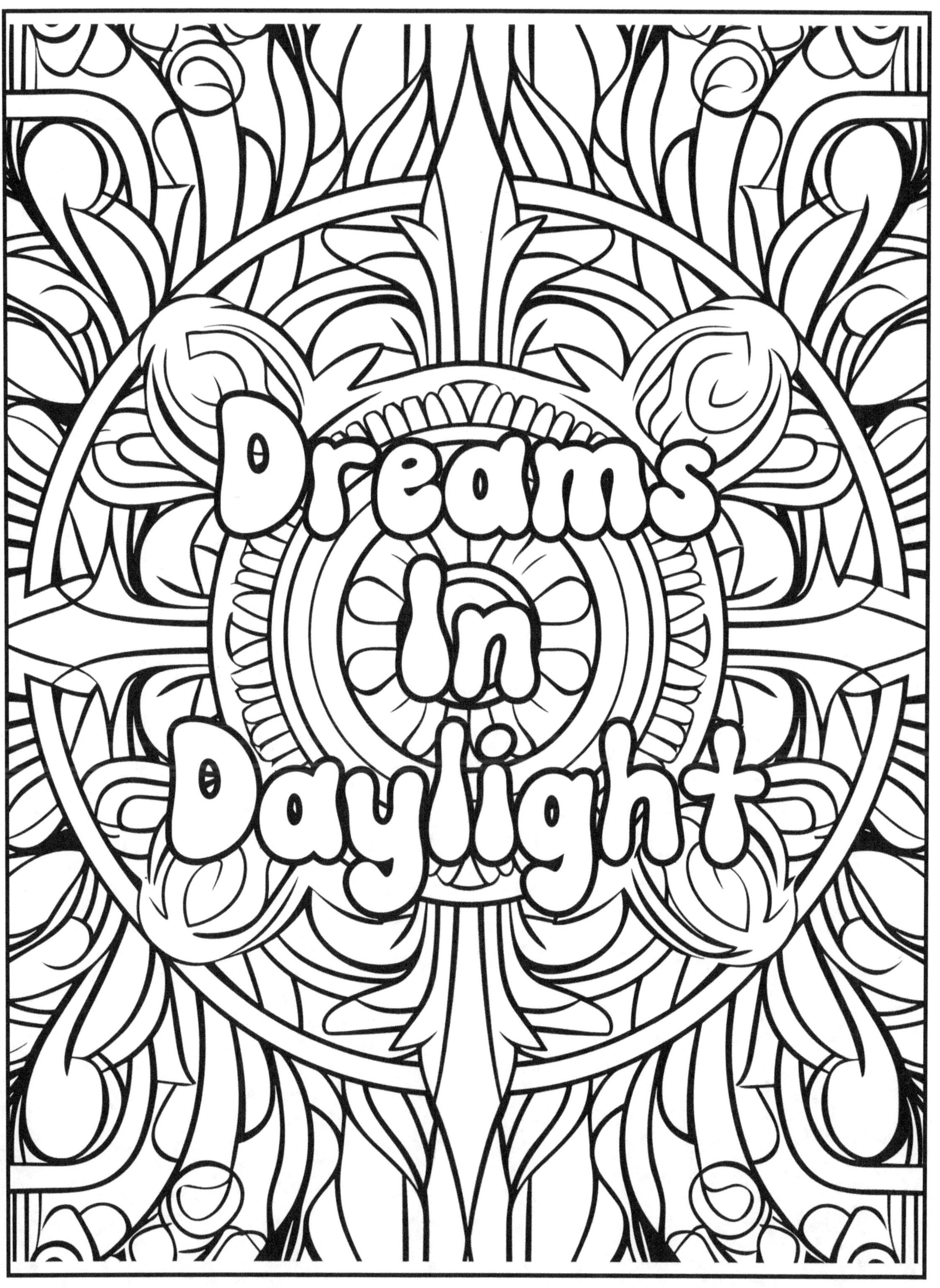
Dreams In Daylight

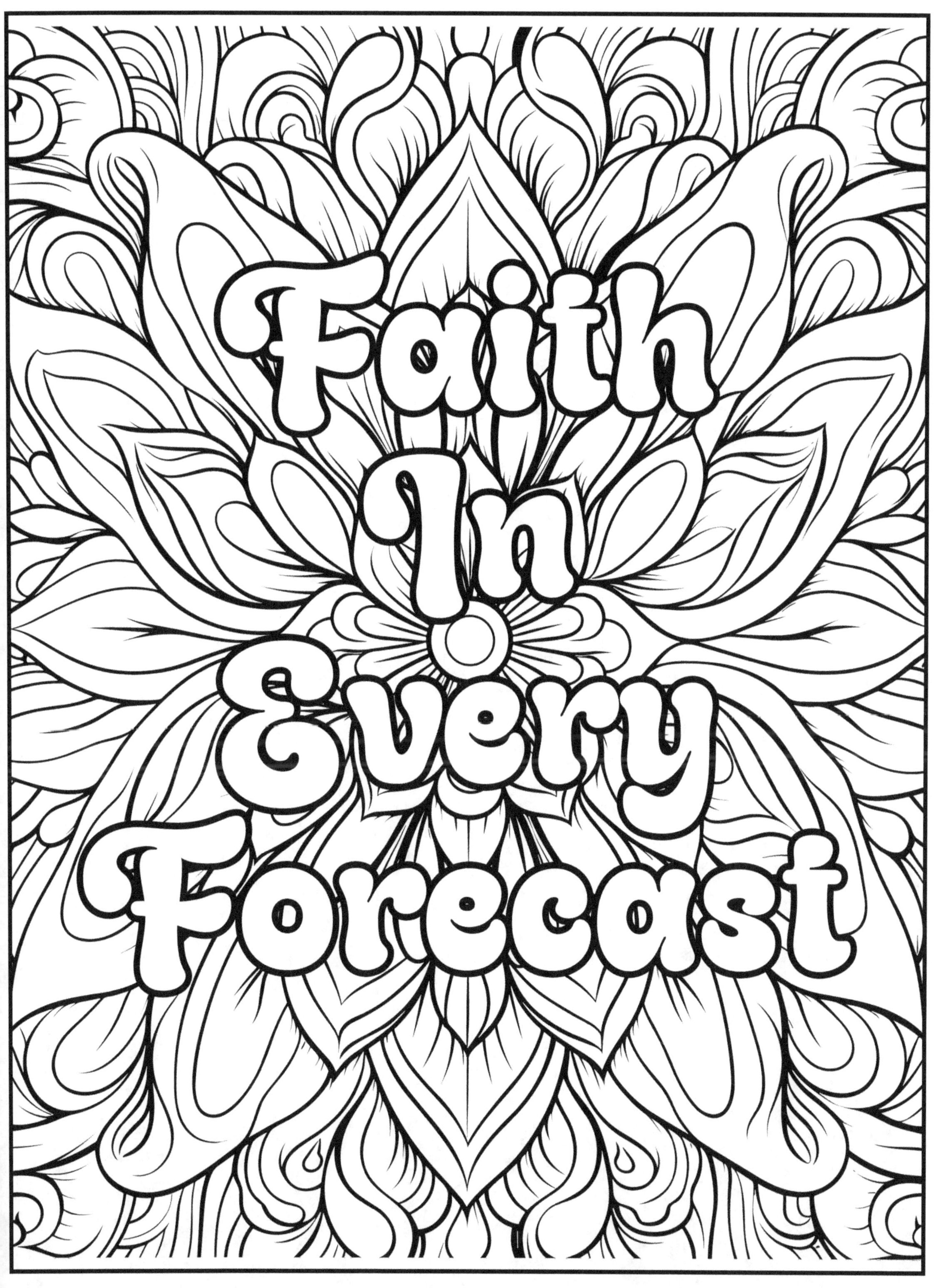

Faith In Every Forecast

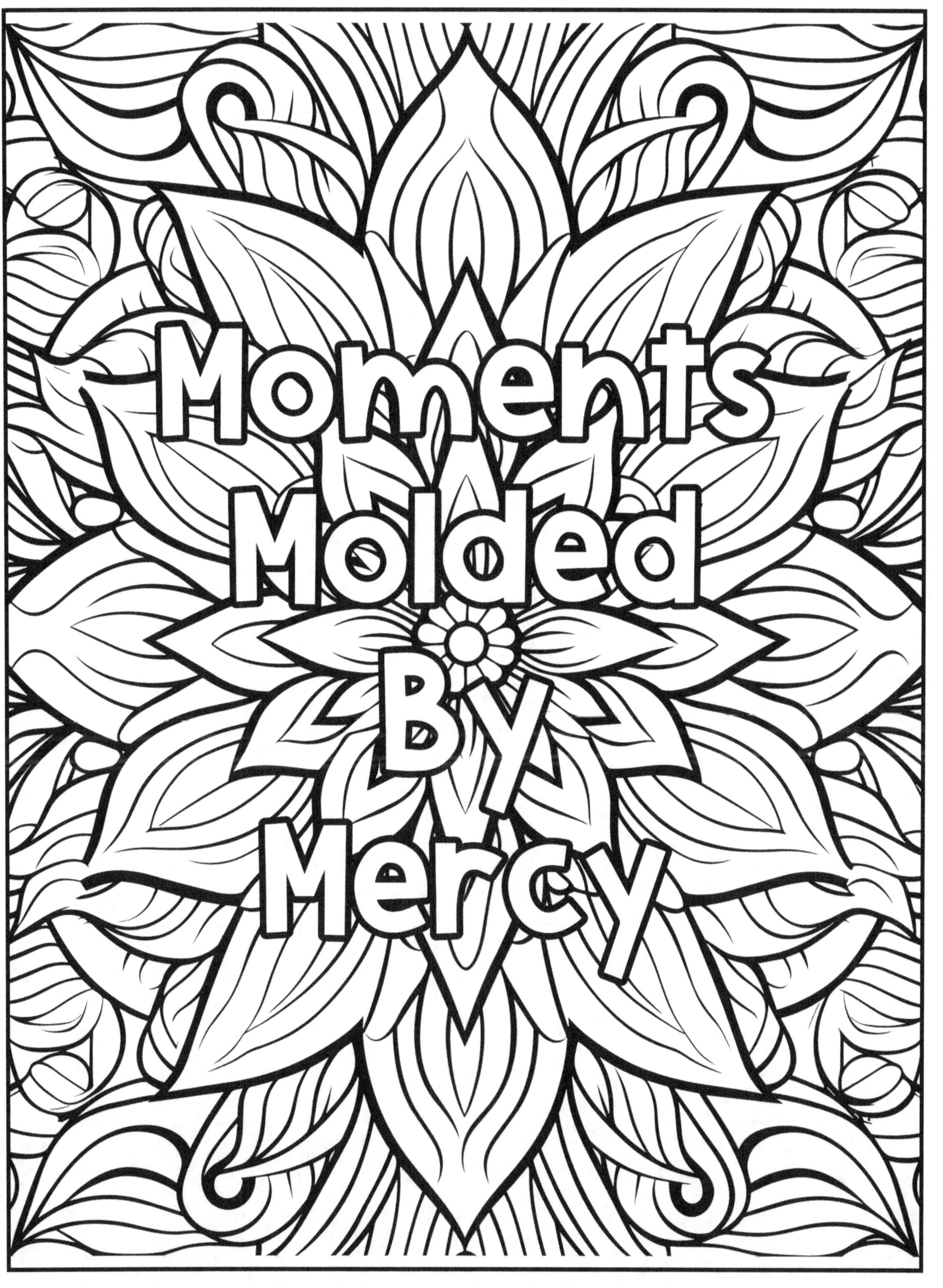

Moments
Molded
By
Mercy

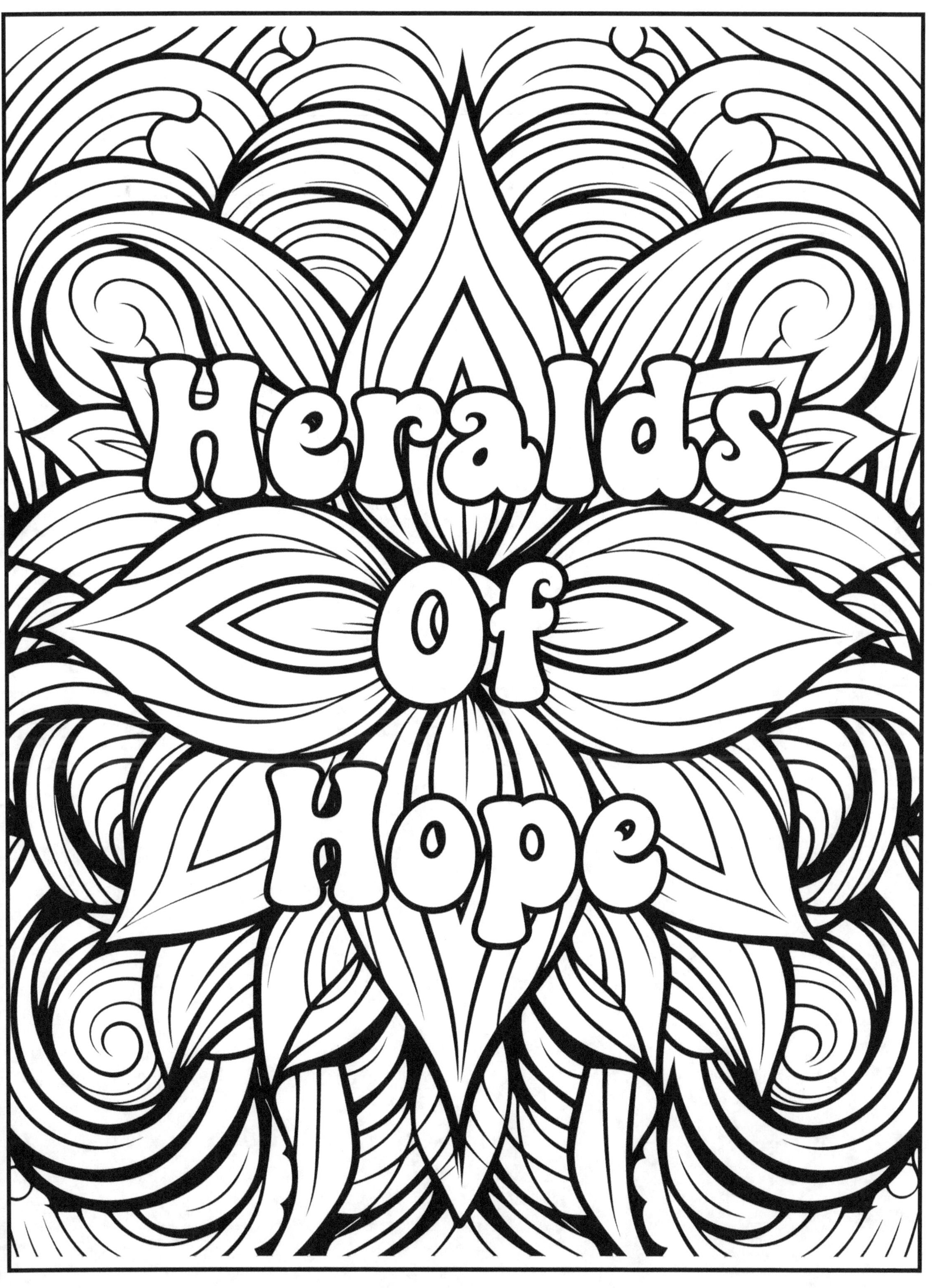

Heralds
Of
Hope

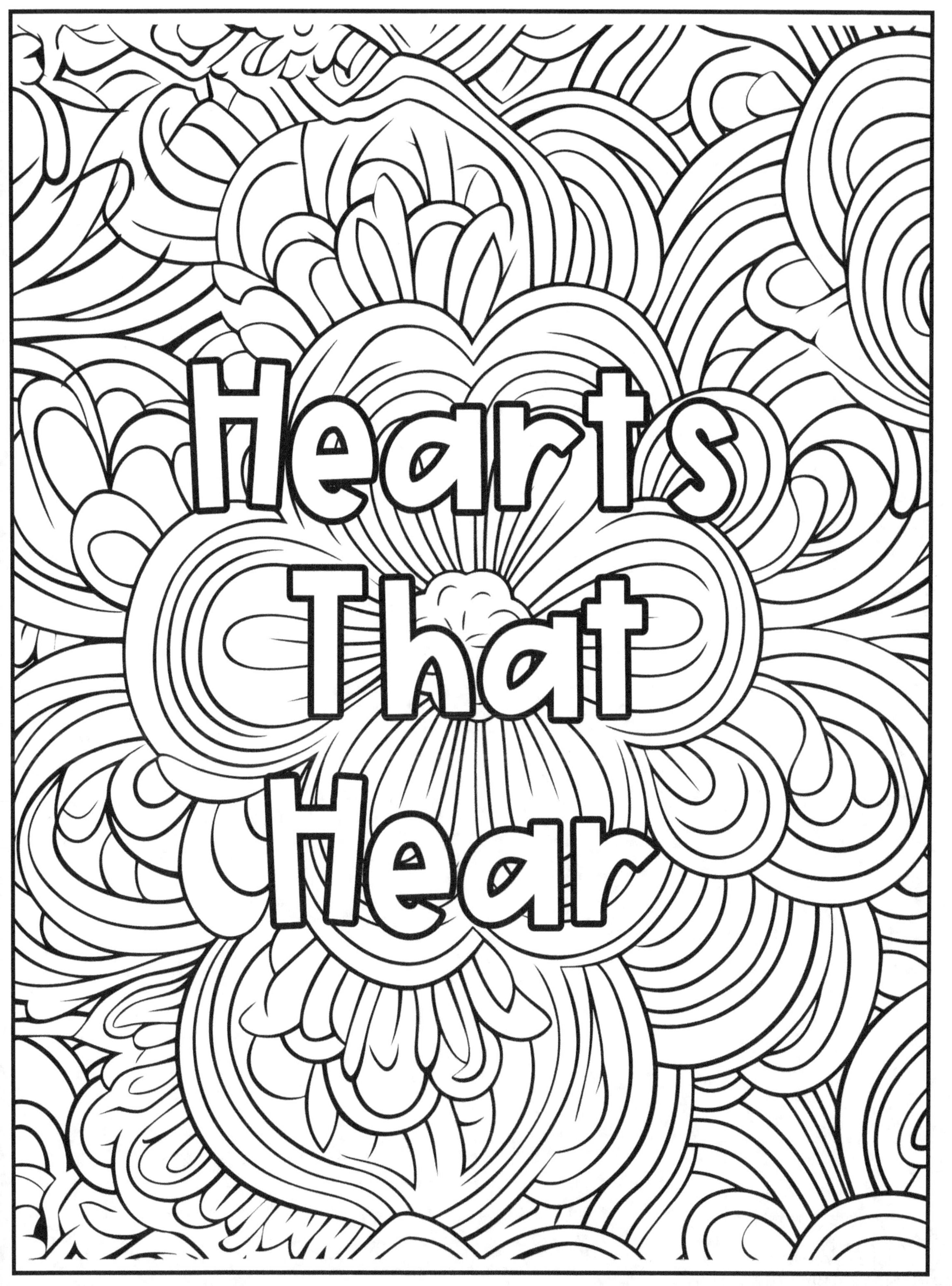

Hearts
That
Hear